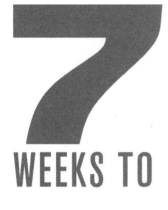

7
WEEKS TO

GETTING RIPPED

D0731202

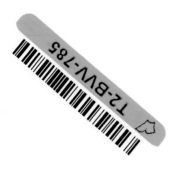

T2-BVV-785

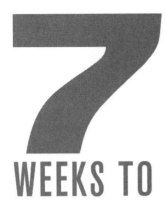

7 WEEKS TO GETTING RIPPED

BRETT STEWART

THE ULTIMATE WEIGHT-FREE, GYM-FREE TRAINING PROGRAM

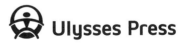

Ulysses Press

This book is dedicated to Dean Karnazes, Timothy Ferriss and Steve Jobs, three men who've inspired me and changed my life in many ways. The first two I have personally thanked for their influence; the last one I unfortunately will never get the chance to thank.

To Vivi and Ian, I love you and am extremely proud of who you are and am very lucky to be your dad.

Published in the United States by
Ulysses Press
P.O. Box 3440
Berkeley, CA 94703
www.ulyssespress.com

ISBN13: 978-1-61243-026-3
Library of Congress Control Number 2011934768

Printed in Canada by Webcom

10 9 8 7 6 5 4 3 2

Acquisitions Editor: Keith Riegert
Managing Editor: Claire Chun
Editor: Lily Chou
Proofreader: Lauren Harrison
Index: Sayre Van Young
Design: whatldesign @ whatweb.com
Interior photographs: © Rapt Productions except page 11 © Kristen Andersen and page 18 © marema/
    shutterstock.com
Cover photographs: © STEEX/istockphoto.com
Models: Evan Clontz, Lauren Harrison, Lewis Elliot, Brett Stewart

Distributed by Publishers Group West

Please Note: This book has been written and published strictly for informational purposes, and in no way should be used as a substitute for consultation with health care professionals. You should not consider educational material herein to be the practice of medicine or to replace consultation with a physician or other medical practitioner. The author and publisher are providing you with information in this work so that you can have the knowledge and can choose, at your own risk, to act on that knowledge. The author and publisher also urge all readers to be aware of their health status and to consult health care professionals before beginning any health program.

CONTENTS

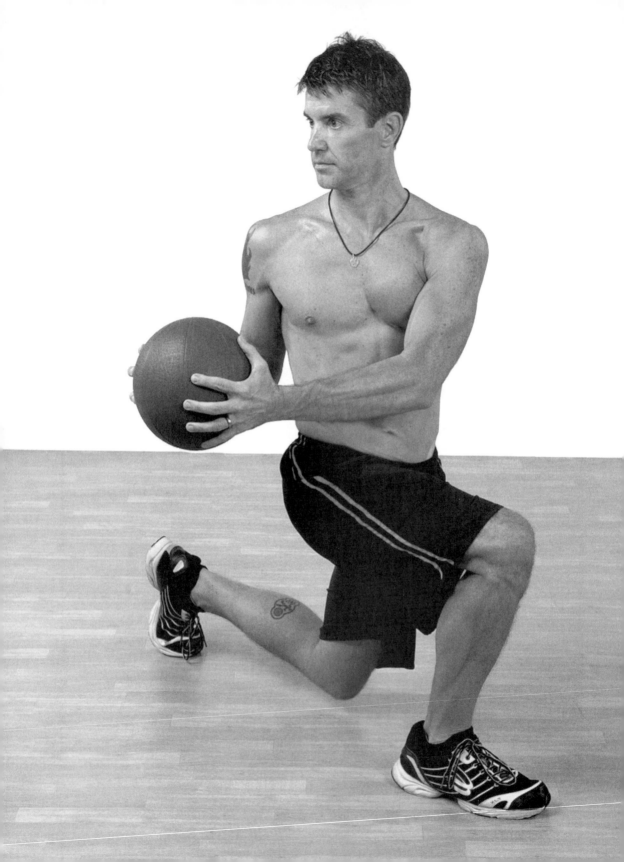

PART 1: OVERVIEW

Introduction

"Jacked," "buff," "built," "cut," "shredded" and "ripped." These are all slang for being in shape—really in shape—the physique that guys and gals alike want to attain. Watch any commercial for weight-loss pills or crazy fitness contraptions and you'll see some dude with six-pack abs, bulging arms and a chiseled chest posing next to a babe with amazing legs, a flat tummy and all the right assets. They smile at the camera and tell you that it's fast, fun and easy to get ripped in just weeks with some incredible diet pill or the BellyRipper2000. You know they're pulling your leg, right? Usually, these models have never even seen the product they're pitching before the video shoot.

So, who do you believe? Should you trust the companies that spend hundreds of thousands of dollars on infomercials? Should you put all your faith in a miracle fat-burning pill? Are you only going to get results if you pay hundreds of dollars a month to a personal trainer?

You know the real answer—it's been there all along and is even easier than you think. Trust your body. Get active, eat healthy and get ripped—that's it.

To most people, building a workout routine is a mystery. Should you do heavy weights and low reps or light weights and high reps? Should you work in supersets or target muscles? Upper body or lower body? Kettlebells, sprints, squats, stairs, pyramids, yadda yadda yadda.

There are more ways to work out than you can count, and they all have their benefits. If you pick up any fitness magazine you'll learn about different "must do" exercises that sometimes conflict with other routines in that same issue! How on earth can you make sense of the information overload and develop an efficient way to get the ripped results you want? Since you're reading this, you no longer have to.

Here's some good news: You can get ripped in as little as seven weeks by following a simple program of easy-to-do

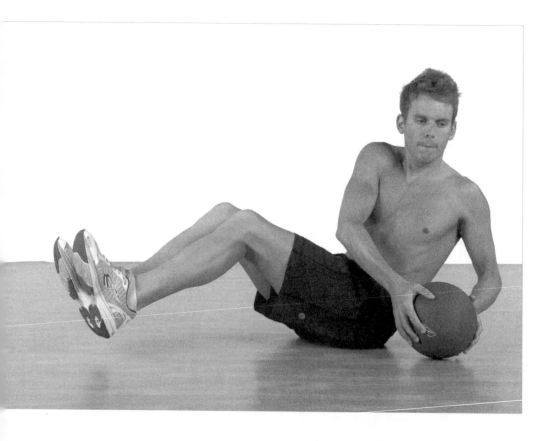

bodyweight exercises and equally simple nutritional guidelines. The even better news is that you don't need any expensive gadgets, a gym membership or even a personal trainer. You're holding in your hands a book devoted to taking the mystery out of getting ripped and showing you step by step how to attain the body you want.

Here's the show-stopping news: *7 Weeks to Getting Ripped* contains "the perfect exercise." That's right, the holy grail of any bodyweight routine—one singular exercise that conditions almost every muscle in your body and shreds your physique like nothing you've ever done before. It's not for the meek, but I can guarantee you won't find it anywhere else, because we invented it. That exercise is called the J-Up and it's hiding out on page 107. (Go ahead and look, I'll hold your place here until you get back.)

The rule of thumb for any lifestyle modification is that it takes anywhere from 7 to 14 days to create a new routine, and this book will make it as easy as possible to get started—and succeed. Your success depends on building a sustainable routine that's familiar, comfortable and repeatable. Working out is hard enough without having to get up early to drive to the gym, remember how to use complicated machines and figure out your daily workout (not to mention locating your membership card!). You can get an incredible full-body workout right in the comfort of your home, saving yourself precious time and gas by not traveling to the gym. You don't even need an expensive rack of dumbbells, bars or how-to DVDs—all you need is your body (you have one of those, right?), a pull-up bar, and maybe a ball or two. We'll get to those later in the games.

Did I mention GAMES? Absolutely. Who said fitness couldn't be fun? Heck, fitness should be fun, otherwise it's just a reason to get tired, sore and sweaty. That's not the way to create a sustainable routine for success and, frankly, it's just not that enjoyable. Don't get me wrong, I like working out (or marathons, triathlons and stuff like that) but if you can have fun and get fit at the same time, why wouldn't you?

How Did I Get Here?

I'm the fat kid in gym class who can't do a single pull-up. I'm the 30-year-old overweight smoker who gets winded walking up a flight of stairs. I'm an Ironman finisher, ultra-marathoner, fitness author and model.

I know what it feels like to be picked last in sports, get laughed at by classmates (and my P.E. teacher) during the Presidential Fitness Test and be complacent about being overweight and unhappy with my appearance. To this day I can vividly remember P.E. in elementary school and my classmate Fran completing countless pull-ups, or playing basketball with Rick and being out of breath after only a few minutes.

I loathed being out of shape and how it held me back in sports, and I envied all my friends who were in great shape. By my mid-20s I had resigned myself to the fact that I'd never be fit like them—and even lied to myself that they were genetically gifted and I wasn't.

The simple truth is I was lazy and never willing to put the effort into being fit. It was much easier to make excuses than it was to put in the work to get control of my diet and get in some structured exercise. But more importantly—I didn't know how to get fit. I avoided gyms because I was embarrassed by my physique, and I didn't have the support structure of really active friends to get me on the right track and keep me motivated. That all changed in the early 2000s when I met the three people who would change my life.

This book isn't a love story, so I'll spare you the details on meeting my wife—but she plays many important roles in my transformation. First off, she detested smoking, so cigarettes were immediately a thing of the past. We met playing softball, and she was very active, fiery and competitive. It didn't take long for her to

inspire those same characteristics in me. Instead of complaining about not being fit, I got competitive with myself and made it my priority to get in shape. Unfortunately, I still didn't know what I was doing. My fitness and weight yo-yoed for the next couple of years and topped out at about 50 pounds overweight at my wedding.

My wedding pictures were a wake-up call, and before my honeymoon was even over, I had made a promise to myself to get lean, fit and ripped—and I had just the friends to do it. I started playing basketball every weekday morning for two hours with Jason (who's about 6" taller than me, so I needed to get faster if I ever hoped to make a basket). Three times a week we'd pick a workout and head outside at lunchtime. We were just guys ripping articles out of health magazines and giving it a shot.

Our workouts got a real upgrade when we met Mike, a certified personal trainer

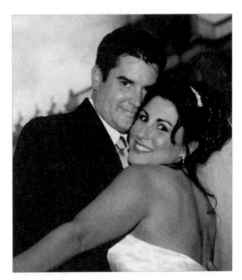

Author Brett Stewart's wedding pictures motivated him to get in shape.

who knew how to get the most out of your body during every workout. Mike pushed us to new limits of fitness while helping us refine our daily workouts. Over the last few years, we started creating different fitness games to compete with each other and keep our workouts fresh—everything from sprinting after a bouncing football on a field to tossing medicine balls as far as we could. Fitness can really be fun if you turn it into a game and share it with your friends.

Jason and Mike are contributors to this book as well as my other book, *7 Weeks to 50 Pull-Ups*. They're the motivating force behind creating the programs for both books as well as being the test subjects and a great source of support.

So, here I am: 40 years old and in the best shape of my life. Over the last six years I've completed over 50 triathlons and even made it to the podium a time or two. I've gone from barely able to run a mile to completing several marathons and ultra-marathons. I'm in the best shape of my life and it's all because I made fitness and balanced nutrition priorities in my life—and this book can help you do exactly the same thing.

Making the Investment

A few years ago I joined a new running group. During my first excursion with them I found myself running next to a guy quite a few years older than me. We made some small talk as we picked up the pace, and as we passed some gorgeous homes he asked me a strange question: "Which property

on this street do you think is the most expensive?"

I looked around for a little bit and admitted I had no idea; real estate wasn't something I know a lot about and all the houses were way out of my price range.

So he tried again: "If you could invest in any property on this road right now, which do you think would give you the most long-term benefit?"

At this point I thought he was a little nuts, so I just randomly picked a house and said, "I guess that one over there."

We ran a few more minutes and I was starting to get quite tired at the rapid pace we were running while his legs still seemed fresh. He slowed down a little bit and got right up next to me and pointed at my chest: "That property right there," he said. "You'll spend more money on that body than any house, car or vacation—invest properly, because it's the only one you'll ever get."

And then the "old guy" left me in his dust.

If you invest in your body, it'll pay you back for years to come.

About the Book

Getting ripped in seven weeks is within your reach, and it'll take balanced nutrition and focused effort on your form in each of the exercises of the progressive routines to achieve your goals. Once you've taken the initial tests to assess your fitness level, this book will guide you through a seven-week program that's sure to help you lose weight, gain strength and muscle definition, and get ripped. If you have the will to succeed and the determination to commit the time and effort, you'll be amazed by the results.

PART I introduces the program, describes how the moves work together to build a ripped physique and presents frequently asked questions, as well as tips and tricks and a primer on balanced nutrition.

PART II contains two different workout routines. *Level 1* is a three-week program for intermediate-level athletes to strengthen and reshape their bodies by building lean muscle and burning fat. *Level 2* is a high-octane four-week program for advanced-level athletes to push their limits while building a super-strong core and developing total-body fitness.

PART III provides step-by-step instruction for all the exercises featured in the program, including the aforementioned "perfect exercise"—the J-Up.

THE APPENDIX contains the Prep-level program, a three-week primer that'll teach you proper form for all the basic moves and build your confidence—and your body—while you prepare for the three- and four-week programs that make up the complete *7 Weeks to Getting Ripped*. The appendix is also where you'll find warm-up and stretching ideas, as well as fitness games.

While this book is an effective way to get into "bikini shape" or to rip up before a vacation or wedding, the reasoning behind the program is to make fitness a part of your life through activity and balanced nutrition. Once you make the change and invest in your fitness, you'll see the payback on every level—more energy, strength, stamina. You'll look fantastic, too! After you've completed the program, you can continue to use this book to either push yourself harder to reach new goals or use the exercises, games and cardio elements to create new routines to maintain your fitness level and physique. Check out "Maintaining Your Ripped Physique" on page 114 for more great ideas.

Why Bodyweight Exercises?

This is a really simple answer: because they work. Your body is the only gym you should ever need. Sure, some gyms have amazing amenities—but you can't take 'em with you. Your body is a lot more portable than a Smith machine, isn't it?

Through balance, stability and mobility, bodyweight exercises also strengthen you in ways that no gym equipment ever can. In order to be "fit," you need to be able to incorporate all the muscles in your body when you squat, twist, reach or jump in sports or everyday life. Strengthening your body by actually using your own bodyweight is natural and involves stimulating muscles through a normal range of motion. Lying flat on a bench or sitting while you pull a bar down are absolutely no match for the full-body strength gains and ripped physique you can get from doing bodyweight exercises with proper form.

Most importantly, using your own bodyweight to get fit is simple, repeatable and always available. It's much easier to sneak in a few sets of bodyweight exercises than it is to pack up and drive to the gym! The more convenient a workout is, the more apt you are to complete it. Throw in some fun and your workouts are downright enjoyable. At the end of the day, the investment of time that you put into bodyweight exercises is so much less than a gym-based workout routine and it's actually more effective at developing total-body fitness. Oh, and better yet, it's free.

Get Ripped While Having Fun: Games & Cardio

When combined with core-shredding games/activities and balanced nutrition, the *7 Weeks to Getting Ripped* program will help develop a lean, ripped body. Games and cardio are an integral part of getting ripped—medicine ball tosses and sprints are an amazing way to burn fat and get fit fast.

The Hot Corner game (page 134) is even better than a boot camp workout because you can do it yourself whenever you want. The most important part about the games and cardio exercises is that

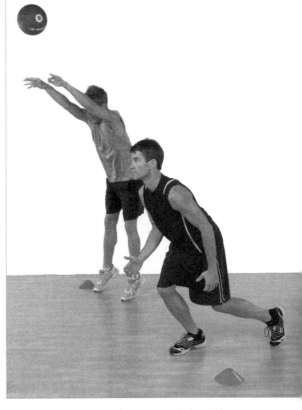

they make the workouts more interesting and fun. We all know that if something is exciting, we're more apt to stick with it, right? The games are also a great way to challenge yourself and your friends; the more support you have, the fewer excuses you have to skip a workout.

RIPPED TIP: The easiest and most effective core exercise you can do is to go outside and get active. Any running, jumping, twisting and lifting will work your core and make your whole body stronger and more fit. The simple truth is every exercise in this book has a positive effect on your core, but in order to develop those sexy rectus abdominis muscles—wait, that doesn't sound sexy at all...how does "six-pack" sound?—you need to isolate and work them. (Truthfully, though, there are four ab muscle pairs for a possible eight-pack.)

The Muscles behind the Movements

The programs and games in *7 Weeks to Getting Ripped* will work all major muscle groups and most ancillary muscles in your body, but instead of covering all 640 muscles, we'll break the body down into two sections: "movers" and "core."

Movers are any muscle whose prime movement is to push, pull or rotate any part of your body aside from your core. The core is the foundation that allows the movers to do their thing and handles twisting and crunching. The stronger your core is, the more effective, efficient and enduring all your mover muscles will be. Building your core strength is the key to total-body fitness and absolutely imperative when developing a fit, ripped physique.

Throughout the book, we'll focus on exercises that use at least one from each group. Most will use both, and at least one exercise will use all of the above. Seriously, it'll use all of them.

Movers

PECTORALIS MAJOR This pair of thick, fan-shaped muscles makes up the bulk of the muscle mass in the chest. The "pecs" are responsible for rotating, flexing and bringing in both arms for actions such as throwing a ball, lifting a child, or performing jumping jacks or push-ups.

TRICEPS BRACHII The large muscle located on the back of the upper arm, the triceps brachii (commonly referred to as "triceps") is responsible for straightening the arm. The triceps makes up over 50 percent of the upper arm's muscular mass.

DELTOID This heart-shaped muscle group is made up of three different fibers (front, middle and rear). While each fiber type has a specific function, the "delts"

as a whole are responsible for raising and stabilizing the arms during rotation.

BICEPS BRACHII One of the assisting muscles during a pull-up, the biceps brachii (commonly referred to as "biceps") is responsible for forearm rotation and elbow flexion. It's located on the front of the upper arm. *Note:* Chin-ups are more effective at targeting the biceps than pull-ups are due to the supinated grip.

TRAPEZIUS Another prime mover, the trapezius (commonly referred to as "traps") is a large, superficial muscle located between the base of the skull and the mid-back, and laterally between both shoulders. Its primary function is to move the scapulae (shoulder blades) and support the arm.

LATISSIMUS DORSI The latissimus dorsi (meaning "broadest muscle in the back") is responsible for moving the arm toward the center of the body (adduction), internally rotating the arm at the shoulder toward the center of the body (medial rotation), and moving the arm straight back behind the body (posterior shoulder extension). It also plays a synergistic role in extending and bending to either side (lateral flexion) the lumbar spine. This pair of muscles is commonly referred to as the "lats."

FOREARM FLEXORS/ EXTENSORS The structure between the elbow and wrist contains a number of muscles, including the flexors and extensors of the digits, brachioradialis

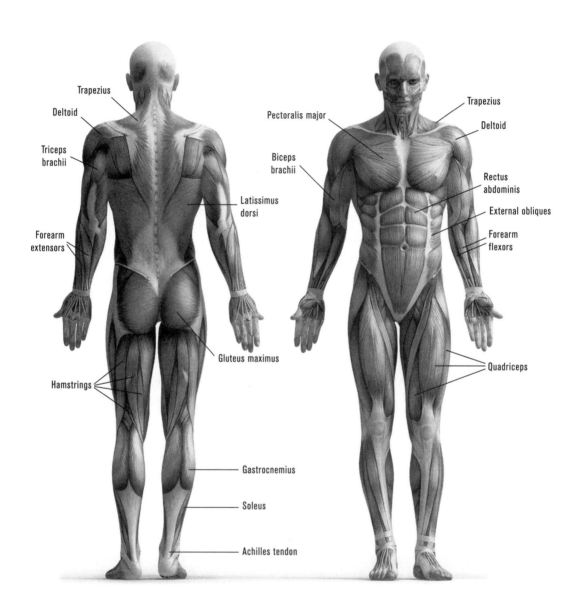

Trapezius

Deltoid

Triceps
brachii

Forearm
extensors

Latissimus
dorsi

Gluteus maximus

Hamstrings

Gastrocnemius

Soleus

Achilles tendon

Pectoralis major

Biceps
brachii

Trapezius

Deltoid

Rectus
abdominis

External obliques

Forearm
flexors

Quadriceps

MAJOR MUSCLES

(which flexes the elbow), pronators (which turn the palm of the hand downward) and supinator (which turns the palm of the hand upward). These muscles allow you to grip the bar during a pull-up.

GLUTEUS MAXIMUS This muscle makes up the majority of the buttocks and is responsible for maintaining an erect posture, raising from a squat position and performing most leg motions, such as adduction and rotation.

QUADRICEPS The quadriceps is a large muscle group made up of four muscles on the front of the thigh. It's the strongest, leanest muscle mass on the body. The "quads" are responsible for straightening the knee joint and are crucial in walking, running, squatting and jumping.

HAMSTRINGS The hamstrings, located on the back of the thigh, are made up of four muscles responsible for knee bending and hip straightening. The hamstrings work as antagonists to the quadriceps to enable walking, running and jumping, as well as maintaining stability in the hip and knee.

CALVES The triceps surae, or "calves," is made up of the gastrocnemius and soleus muscles. These muscles attach to the Achilles tendon and are responsible for ankle rotation, flexion and stabilization, and are crucial for walking, running and jumping.

Core

This term refers to the area of the torso composed of the rectus abdominis (the "six-pack" portion of the abdominals), obliques, transversus abdominis and erector spinae. Full-body functional movements traditionally originate from this area of the body, and it provides stabilization during pretty much every activity your body performs on a daily basis, from exercises including the pull-up to maintaining proper posture when standing or sitting. A strong core is essential to proper fitness; your body's strength needs a solid base to work from.

5-SECOND ABS
To work your core in the car, the office, in a dentist's chair and everywhere in between, practice flexing your rectus abdominis like you're about to get punched in the gut. Breathe out and hold each contraction for 3–5 seconds for as many reps as you can—until your dental hygienist starts wondering what the heck you're doing. Doing this quick isometric exercise can keep your body working to shred your core in between workouts. It's simple and you don't even have to change into your stinky gym clothes.

Frequently Asked Questions

Q. Is it possible to just work off my love handles?

A. Yes, but the answer might be different than you think. The secret to losing your love handles is to train your entire body using bodyweight exercises. Want ripped abs? Train your arms, back, shoulders and legs…and your abs will reap the benefits.

Q. Can't I just do crunches to rip my abs?

A. You can do crunches all day long and still not have a ripped core. Period. Unless you work your entire body to get lean, you just won't be able to show off your six-pack.

Q. I was always told to stretch first, but lately I've read that you shouldn't stretch your muscles when you're cold. What's the deal?

A. Research and studies over the last few years have reinforced the reasoning that you should warm up before you exercise and then stretch after you've completed your workout. Read more about warming up and stretching on page 30.

Q. Isn't it true that bodyweight exercises don't make your muscles as big as gym-based exercises?

A. If you want to build the biggest chest possible by loading up a bar and doing reps of bench press over and over, this is probably the wrong book for you. But remember, you can build huge arms, pecs and legs and still be unfit—unable to perform well at the complex motions necessary for most sports. Using bodyweight exercises, you'll build your entire body and the end result will be a stronger, faster and fitter version of you. You'll also be amazed at how much bigger muscles look when you're ripped.

Q. Can I do a full-body workout every day?

A. No, your body needs time to rest and recover. When you do strength-training exercises such as pull-ups, you create tiny, harmless tears in the muscle. These tiny tears heal during rest days. As a result, the muscle becomes stronger and more defined. If you don't allow the muscles to heal, you risk overuse injuries that could potentially derail your ability to exercise at all. Constant repetitions of any motion without proper rest will eventually result in overuse injuries. Repeat this sentence: "Rest is equally as important as the workout for strengthening and shredding your body." Now, make sure you follow your own advice.

Q. What if I can't do all the reps in the program for a given workout?

A. The reps are a guideline and a goal for each workout—they're not the law. I can promise you that no one will show up at your door to give you a ticket for missing the last two reps of pull-ups. Do as many reps as you can with good form and when you reach failure, your body is signaling that you're done. If you still feel like you have some fuel left in the tank, then take a break for 1–2 minutes and try to finish off the set. If you feel any pain, soreness or dizziness, then it's time to call it a day. Never feel ashamed that you didn't complete every rep of a workout—stay positive and come back strong after a day of rest.

If you missed more than 30 percent of the reps, I suggest starting over the same workout after you've rested and recovered. Feel free to progress onward if it's just one or two reps, but be honest with yourself if you find yourself missing reps every workout—perform the exercises within your ability and you'll get stronger and eventually be able to complete the full workout.

Q. How fast should I do the movements?

A. Some exercises will have specific speeds during certain workouts, but as a rule of thumb you should try to stick to a "medium" speed. Listen to your body; you'll know what's too fast or too slow with a little bit of experience. If you're just learning the movements, take it as slowly as you need to maintain proper form. A few exercises like sprints and Tabatas will require 90 percent effort and speed, but we'll get to those when we cover the program.

Q. How should I breathe for each movement?

A. For most exercises we'll cover when to breathe in and out, but overall it's a good idea to breathe out when you're exerting the most force (pushing, pulling, etc.) and breathe in on the recovery. Breathing properly is a big part of being able to perform some of the rapid movements we'll be covering on in this book, so make sure to focus on breathing rhythmically and not holding your breath during sets.

Q. I was able to follow the program very well early on but am now having trouble doing the required reps. What's going on?

A. Initially, your body goes through a number of changes when you start a new program. Your body will soon begin to adapt to the workouts; you'll notice a plateau once you become used to doing any exercise. This program has been carefully designed to avoid this plateau effect by changing the duration, intensity and workout routine over seven weeks. Follow the program as best you can. In the unlikely event you do hit a plateau, continue to follow the plan and eventually there'll be enough change to get you over the hump. Remember, don't overdo it and be sure to take the necessary rest between workouts.

Q. Should I be sore after every workout?

A. Soreness may be normal if you're a beginner, have recently changed up your routine or are trying a new activity. The initial soreness should lessen over time; it's not normal to be sore after every workout. If you continue to be sore, you may need to take more days off between workouts.

Q. Will full-body strength training make women bulk up?

A. The bodyweight exercises in this book were selected specifically for men and women to develop lean, shredded bodies. Typically, women don't have the kind of hormones necessary to build huge, bulky muscles. Full-body strength training benefits both men and women by creating leaner tissue and losing any excess fat (by increasing metabolic efficiency), slowing muscle loss (especially in older adults) and decreasing risk for injury.

Q. Will this workout be an effective way to lose weight?

A. The combination of bodyweight strength training with the cardiovascular training from performing supersets (many exercises with no rest in between), Tabatas (20 seconds of intense exercise followed by 10 seconds of rest) and the sprinting involved in the fitness games is the most

efficient way for you to lose weight. When paired with balanced nutrition, you'll be firing up your metabolism in as little as 20 minutes a day to burn excess fat and shred your physique.

Q. What is the best time of day to do these workouts?

A. Choosing a time is completely up to your preference. I personally like the feeling of a great morning routine energizing me for the whole day, but I originally conceived this program while working out at lunchtime at the park near my office. After a quick shower at the gym, I was more energized at work in the

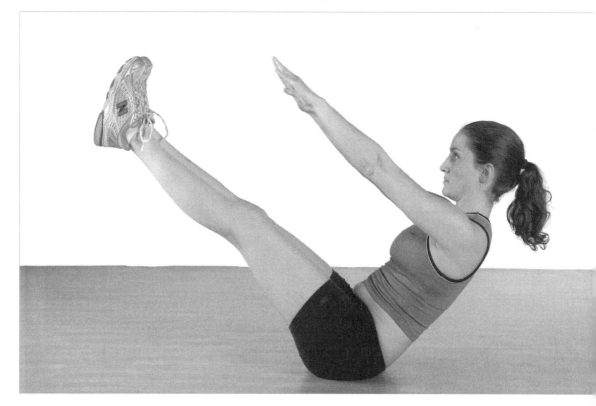

afternoon after workouts than I was in the morning. The workouts in this book are designed to be done almost anywhere, so pick a time that works for you. You could do sets of exercises while you get ready in the morning or after you get the kids to bed.

Q. Can I combine other workouts with this program?

A. If you're an athlete who needs to train sports-specific skills, then the workouts in this book should be used to supplement that training. If you're hoping to get stronger or more ripped faster by doing extra workouts on "rest days," then you're in danger of overtraining and not letting your muscles rest, recover and grow. For best results, follow the program—rest included—for seven weeks. If you're doing the program for maintenance, check out the advice in the "Maintaining Your Ripped Physique" section on page 114.

Q. How do I use the games to help me get ripped?

A. All of the games are secretly fantastic workouts to shred your body and can be done in place of the cardio component (medicine ball sprints are a great example) on workout days or as a supplemental weekend workout. Fun, tough and guaranteed to get you sweating, these games have been tested and created over the course of several years and were instrumental in my cross-training in preparation for racing my first Ironman.

Q. What's the single best tip you can give to someone about to start this program?

A. Commit the time and effort to do the program right. Often it really helps to have a partner or two (that's how we created the programs!) who'll keep you on track to complete the workouts. Mark workout days on your calendar, or set an alert on your computer or smartphone for the short amount of time the program takes. You can do what Jason and I did—block your calendar from noon to 1 p.m. each day to make sure you get uninterrupted exercise time.

Balanced Nutrition

Balanced nutrition is actually pretty simple, but we're bombarded by millions of dollars worth of advertising touting unhealthy foods. For the most part, we spend very little time really thinking about what we put into our mouths on a daily basis. Sure, we're all busy every day, but a little planning and picking up some healthy snacks can prevent your stomach from steering you into a really unhealthy food choice.

Developing balanced nutrition just requires a little knowledge of your food's nutritional value and some easy planning. Your body constantly adjusts to stay in balance. It may sound like a ridiculous oversimplification but, by eating healthy, balanced foods, you make it that much easier for your body to function at peak condition. Here are my top-10 superquick tips for assessing your daily food intake.

TIP 1: KEEP A FOOD JOURNAL FOR A WEEK.

Write down absolutely everything that you put in your belly—water included—for seven days (or longer, if necessary) so you can figure out your patterns. Include time, quantity and how hungry you felt on a scale of 1–10. Make a note about what physical activity you did that day as well; there's usually a correlation between exertion and hunger. The more information you put in your journal, the more data you have to analyze and figure out your patterns.

TIP 2: DON'T LET YOURSELF GET FAMISHED.

If your stomach is grumbling, there's a good chance you'll overeat or snack on something unhealthy. You're more prone to ignore the unhealthiness of your snack or overdo the portions in your impulse to fill your belly. Eating smaller meals more often throughout the day is the easiest way to combat the tummy grumbles and avoid sabotaging your daily food intake.

TIP 3: SPEND MORE TIME IN THE PRODUCE AISLE OF YOUR GROCERY STORE.

Fresh veggies require a little more effort than grabbing french fries at a drive-through, but one builds healthy bodies and the other builds love handles. Experiment with adding a green pepper to your morning omelet in place of bacon or have an apple instead of a candy bar.

RIPPED TIP: Shop at the edges of the grocery store. Grocery stores generally keep products that spoil (i.e., have no artificial preservatives) at the exterior edges of the store, leaving the interior for canned goods, processed foods and boxed items. Watch where you're spending the majority of your time and where you're getting the bulk of your calories. General rule: If you get most of your calories from the interior of a grocery store, you need to change your diet.

TIP 4: TAKE A PICTURE OF YOUR FOOD AND DRINK BEFORE YOU EAT IT.

This helps you remember what you ate, when you ate it and the portion size. Often, when you're really hungry, you overlook all the extra calories in that meal—the cheese, condiments, bacon, etc. If your food came in a package that has a label, take a picture of that, too. Balanced nutrition starts with knowing the nutritional value of your food. Use those labels to help with planning your protein, carbohydrate, fat and calorie intake.

TIP 5: DRINK MORE WATER.

Soda pop, lemonade, energy drinks, beer—they taste so good and are a huge part of our daily lives. Unfortunately, they're also a huge part of our daily *caloric intake*. A quick web search shows that the average American consumes approximately 400 calories a day from sugary beverages. Those 146,000 extra calories can translate into as much as 40 pounds of weight gain a year. Here's the great news: If you cut sugary drinks out of your daily fluid intake and drink 2–3 quarts of ice cold water a day, you'll benefit from:

- Cutting hundreds of calories (and chemicals) from your daily intake.

- Burning more calories (part I)—ice cold water makes your body work harder to warm it to body temperature.

- Burning more calories (part II)—the more hydrated you are, the more often you'll urinate. Each trip to the restroom will force you to get up from your desk and be active.

- Regulating your blood pressure, transporting nutrients and keeping all your bodily systems running smoothly.

RIPPED TIP: "Protein" rhymes with "lean." While the USDA RDA for protein is .36 grams per pound of bodyweight to maintain a healthy diet, to get ripped you need to consume approximately 1 gram of lean protein per pound of your desired weight. In order to do this, you'll need to plan your meals and snacks around protein content first, and these lean proteins will make up about 50% of your daily food intake. See "Eating to Get—and Stay—Ripped" on page 115 for more information.

TIP 6: EAT REAL FOODS.

The more you can avoid processed foods, the healthier you'll be. Meat, fish, poultry, vegetables, fruits, nuts and seeds don't have nutrition facts labels on them because you know what nutritional value they contain. While I'm not advocating a full-on diet change, the Paleo diets are very effective in helping some individuals get healthier and lean. I suggest meeting in the middle—fewer processed foods than you eat now and more healthier real foods. If you're vegetarian or gluten intolerant, you'll need to adjust any food intake to meet your dietary restrictions.

TIP 7: AVOID THE EXTRA CALORIES WHEN EATING OUT.

When you're eating at home, you know exactly what ingredients are going into your meal. When eating out, you have a lot less knowledge of and control over all the extra calories that get put into that meal. The added butter, salt, sugar and dressing can really add up to make that healthy meal you ordered a calorie and fat bomb. Ask for any dressing on the side and your meats or vegetable cooked "plain" without sauces or butter. Spend a few minutes scanning the menu for healthy choices and make sure to ask your server to help keep them healthy. It's really that simple. If you can't find a healthy choice, then choose a salad with plenty of veggies (and even some grilled chicken) and make sure you get the dressing on the side. Sometimes it's better to have a salad, leave a little hungry and have a healthy snack at home.

TIP 8: WHAT HAPPENS IN THE PANTRY DOESN'T STAY IN THE PANTRY.

The first step is to banish all the unhealthy snack food from your house—if it's not there, you can't snack on it. Sure, you may have fantastic willpower, but when you have a craving and see that bag of chips, you're putting yourself in a predicament for no good reason. Having some fruit in a bowl on the counter works wonders—you see it constantly, you can grab it on the way out the door and you'll also feel guilty if you bought it and allowed it to go bad right under your nose. Celery and carrots last even longer in the fridge than fruit and are always a great snack. A handful of nuts and dried cranberries will go a long way in fueling your body and fending off any cravings for sugary snacks.

RIPPED TIP: Stock your fridge, have a sparse pantry. As a corollary to shopping at the exterior edges of the grocery store, take inventory of your fridge and pantry. The majority of your calories should come from the fridge and freezer rather than the pantry.

TIP 9: PLAN YOUR SNACKS JUST LIKE YOUR MEALS.

A "snack" absolutely does not have to be something decadent that you need to feel bad about after eating. Actually, snacks play a major role in fueling your body throughout the day. Did you know that your body burns more calories while it's processing food than when you have an empty stomach? Snacks fill in the gap between meals and keep your body burning calories all day long. Plan your snacks by bringing a couple of pieces of fruit to work or on your daily activities. Granola, nuts and dried fruit all travel well. There are plenty of healthy options in energy and nutrition bars, but be aware of the calorie density and nutritional value. If you're (occasionally) eating a meal-replacement bar, make sure it's replacing a meal and not a snack. If you have healthy snacks available, you'll make your choices far more easily.

TIP 10: IT'S ALL ABOUT BALANCE.

In order to stay active, build a lean physique, and keep your energy level high, you need to get enough macro- and micronutrients and water each day. Macronutrients include fats, proteins and carbohydrates; micronutrients include vitamins and minerals. Your body requires vitamins to regulate its complex chemistry, including that of the digestive and nervous systems. Minerals are the building blocks for bone strength and cardiovascular health. Meats, fruits and vegetables contain plenty of the vitamins and minerals your body needs on a daily basis. Vitamin supplements are also a good way to make sure your body is getting the vital micronutrients it needs.

Before You Begin

In order to focus on completing this program successfully, it's important to be ready for the challenge and know your limits. When you begin any new exercise program, it's imperative that you talk with your doctor first and make sure you're healthy enough to participate in physical strength training and conditioning.

Once you begin the *7 Weeks to Getting Ripped* program, perform it at your own pace and within your personal level of fitness. If you feel extremely fatigued or have an uncomfortable level of pain and soreness, take two to three days off from the workout. If the discomfort or pain persists, you should see a health care professional.

Due to the nature of a full-body workout routine, you'll be lifting, pushing and pressing your entire bodyweight. Make sure you recognize any physical limitations such as weak or injury-prone joints. It's far more important to be careful with nagging injuries than it is to be worry about completing all the exercises in a specified amount of time. Seven weeks is an optimum amount of time to get ripped, but not if you ignore the warning signs and hurt yourself.

Some moves will require you to lift your bodyweight on bars, benches, chairs or other objects. Please make sure that the apparatus you're using is sturdy enough to handle more than double your weight. Be smart and safe—don't take any chances with unsafe equipment, and make sure you're properly trained to use any equipment before you start a workout. Always be aware of your surroundings and make sure you have plenty of room to execute moves safely without hitting or tripping over other objects.

Warming Up & Stretching

Properly warming up the body prior to any activity is very important, as is stretching post-workout. Please note that warming up and stretching are two completely different things: A warm-up routine should be done before stretching so that your muscles are more pliable and able to be stretched efficiently. You should not "warm up" by stretching; you simply don't want to push, pull or stretch cold muscles.

Prior to warming up, your muscles are significantly less flexible. Think of pulling a rubber band out of a freezer: If you stretch it forcefully before it has a chance to warm up, you'll likely tear it. Stretching cold muscles can cause a significantly higher rate of muscle strains and even injuries to joints that rely on those muscles for alignment.

It's crucial to raise your body temperature prior to beginning a workout. In order to prevent injury, such as a muscle strain, you want to loosen up your muscles and joints before you begin the actual exercise movement. A good warm-up before your workout should slowly raise your core body temperature, heart rate and breathing. Before jumping into the workout, you must increase blood flow to all working areas of the body. This augmented blood flow will transport more oxygen and nutrients to the muscles being worked. The warm-up will also increase the range of motion of your joints.

Another goal is to focus your mental awareness and body proprioception. You've heard that meditation requires being present in the "now." The same is true for a demanding exercise routine. Being totally present and focused will help you perform better and avoid injury.

A warm-up should consist of light physical activity (such as walking, jogging, stationary biking or jumping jacks) and only take 5–10 minutes to complete. Your individual fitness level and the activity determine how hard and how long you should go but, generally speaking, the average person should build up to a light sweat during warm-ups. You want to prepare your body for activity, not fatigue it.

A warm-up should be done in these stages:

- **GENTLE MOBILITY:** Easy movements that get your joints moving freely, like standing arm raises, arm and shoulder circles, neck rotations, and trunk twists.

- **PULSE RAISING:** Gentle, progressive, aerobic activity that starts the process of raising your heart rate, like jumping jacks, skipping rope or running in place.

- **SPECIFIC MOBILITY:** This begins working the joints and muscles that will be used during the activity. Perform dynamic movements to prepare your body for your upcoming full-body workout. These movements are done more rapidly than the gentle mobility movements—envision a swimmer before a race or a weightlifter before a big lift. Dynamic movements should raise the heart rate, loosen specific joints and muscles, and get you motivated for your workout.

Stretching should generally be done after a workout. It'll help you reduce soreness from the workout, increase range of motion and flexibility within a joint or muscle, and prepare your body for any future workouts. Stretching immediately post-exercise while your muscles are still warm allows your muscles to return to their full range of motion (which gives you more flexibility gains) and reduces the chance of injury or fatigue in the hours or days after an intense workout. It's important to remember that even when you're warm and loose, you should never "bounce" during stretching. Keep your movements slow and controlled.

To recap, you should warm up for 5–10 minutes, perform your workout, and then stretch for 5–10 minutes. We've included a few warm-up exercises and stretches that specifically target the muscles used in each workout (see page 116).

Avoiding Injuries

As I covered earlier in the FAQs (page 20), bodyweight strength training combined with cardiovascular exercises is the most efficient way to build strength and develop a lean, ripped physique. Let's be honest, though; none of us is perfect. Due to years of improper posture, sports injuries or even weak musculature, we all have imbalances that can affect proper form and even put us on the fast track to injury. In addition, jumping into a new exercise routine too quickly or doing the exercises with improper form can exacerbate any pre-existing injury.

It's very important that you focus on proper form and utilize the proper muscles to complete each exercise. This means no cheating by arching your back on push-ups or swinging your legs on pull-ups. You're only cheating yourself; every proper form rep just gets you closer to ripped! If you have a pre-existing condition like rotator cuff soreness or a muscular imbalance, take your time and work your way up slowly while focusing on training with good form. If pain or soreness persists, please see a medical professional.

Speaking of professionals, remember that no one expects you to be a pro at every movement. Some exercises may come naturally while others feel completely foreign. I personally fight with keeping my shoulders level when performing pull-ups. All you can do is keep working on perfecting the form and get stronger along the way. Don't give up and sit out an exercise if you can't do it—make the investment in yourself and learn the proper form for each move. You'll only reap the benefits.

Listen to Your Body

You should be able to tell when you're ready to begin a strength and conditioning program like this one by tuning in to your body. Take it easy and be smart about determining what's normal soreness from a workout and what's a nagging injury that you're aggravating. If you think it's the latter, take a few extra days off and see if the soreness passes. If it doesn't, you should see a medical professional.

Throughout the routine, you should expect to experience mild soreness and fatigue, especially when you're just getting started. The feeling of your muscles being "pumped" and the fatigue of an exhausting workout should be expected. These are positive feelings.

On the other hand, any sharp pain, muscle spasm or numbness is a warning sign that you need to stop and not push yourself any harder. Some small muscle groups may fatigue more quickly because they're often overlooked in other workouts. Your hands and forearms are doing a tremendous amount of work and can easily tire out. If you feel you can't grip or support yourself with your hands anymore, take a rest. It's far better than slipping and getting hurt.

Here are a few other symptoms to watch for: sore elbows, shoulder (rotator cuff) pain and stiff neck. Sore elbows are usually a sign that you're locking out your elbows when your arms are fully extended; remember to keep a slight bend in your elbows. Pain in the rotator cuff can be caused by poor form or a hand position that is too wide while doing pull-ups or push-ups. A stiff neck can result from straining your neck throughout the movement; try to keep your neck loose and flexible. If any of these pains persists, it's imperative that you seek medical advice.

How to Use This Book

Designed for men and women to build total-body strength and fitness, the *7 Weeks to Getting Ripped* program puts together bodyweight exercises, games, warm-ups, stretches and cardiovascular routines for a unique workout. It also produces results that you need to see—and feel—to believe. The program is broken down into three levels: Prep, Level I and Level II.

The Prep level makes the program accessible to anyone who's interested in getting ripped, regardless of age, weight or fitness level. This level will build your strength and confidence by teaching you full-body exercises that are easy to remember and repeat.

Level I is the meat and potatoes of the program, with carefully chosen exercises to help you develop lean muscle and burn fat.

Level II kicks things up a notch by integrating Tabata intervals, advanced moves and an additional set or two. Level II will keep you on your toes and work your entire body like no other workout you'll find!

How do you find out where you start in the *7 Weeks to Getting Ripped* program? Take the "Power 4" test on page 36!

Find Your Level Using the "Power 4" Exercises

The "Power 4" test measures your ability to perform four exercises: pull-ups, squats, push-ups and planks. You'll do the maximum amount of each of these with good form, followed by a two-minute break.

What? You want me to do all these exercises back to back? I can't do as many push-ups after my upper body is tired from pull-ups!

Yes, that's the whole idea. Throughout Level I and Level II of the program, you'll be performing different intervals, including supersets (completing exercises with little or no rest between sets or movements) and Tabata intervals (20 seconds of intense exercise followed by 10 seconds of rest, then repeated up to 8 times). By "semi-supersetting" (2-minute rest in between exercises), this test closely mirrors the actual workouts and will give you an accurate baseline.

If you're unsure about tackling these exercises by yourself, why not invite a friend to take on this challenge with you? Having a training partner is a great way to keep you safe, motivated and accountable for your workouts. If you have a training partner for the initial test, have them keep an eye on your form to make sure you're performing the movement properly. If you're having problems with your form, now is the easiest time to fix it.

Incorporating Games & Cardio

What about the games and cardio, you ask? The games and cardio exercises are all listed in the Appendix starting on page 126; for the most part they're all mix and match. If your workout calls for 15 minutes of cardio afterward, then you can pick any cardio or game from the list and put in at least 15 minutes of quality exercise. Whether you hop on the treadmill and do "music intervals" or hit a patch of grass for ball sprints, the routine is up to you. You can even combine two or three cardio exercises and games to allow a wide range of motion and get your metabolism fired up.

Some games are a complete workout by themselves and a great way to get outside and get some extra training in on the weekend. "Hot Corner" (page 134) features bodyweight exercises, sprints and dynamic moves that'll keep you moving over the weekend and is a fantastic way for you to include your family and friends in some healthy competition.

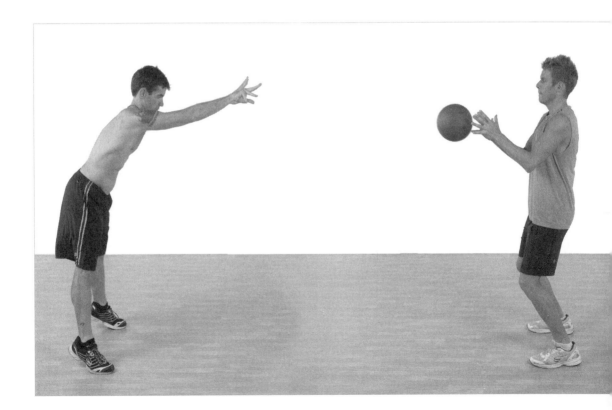

"Power 4" Test

Before beginning the test, it's imperative that you prepare yourself for the exercises by warming up and getting your blood pumping. A good warm-up should be 5-10 minutes and raise your body temperature to a light sweat. Flip to pages 116–21 for some ideas.

Here's what you'll need for the test:

- Pull-up bar
- Stopwatch/timer for planks
- Water
- Towel
- Exercise mat (preferred, but optional)

Your workout area should be well-ventilated and free from obstructions so you can complete the movements freely without hitting anything. Use an appropriate bar that's high enough that you can extend your arms fully when grasping it. If it's too high, you may feel uncomfortable jumping up to grab it. If it's too low, you'll waste energy bending your knees to keep your feet from touching the ground. The bar itself should be safe and sturdy and able to hold more than double your bodyweight.

Warmed up and ready? Great! Just a few minutes more and you can start the test. Before you do, it's very important that you familiarize yourself with proper form for each exercise. Read each of the exercise descriptions, view the photos and slowly try each move yourself a few times to make sure you understand exactly what you'll be doing once you get started.

Make sure you're hydrated, somewhat relaxed and take some slow, deep breaths to prepare. We're starting with the most difficult of the "Power 4" moves—the pull-up. Even if you've never been able to do a pull-up in the past, it's important that you try. I've personally witnessed many people who thought they couldn't do any do 3 or 4 once they realize the proper form and use the large muscles of their upper back to complete the movement. Don't mentally block yourself from success; give it your best shot.

RIPPED TIP: Take a "before" picture. Actually, take several from different angles. Guys, take your shirts off, and ladies, pick that bikini that you'd love to look great in. This is a really important step that is often forgotten and best taken care of before you even take the test. Personally, I wish I had some good shirt-off "before" pictures of myself. Truth be told, I never took any shirtless pictures because I was unhappy with the way I looked. Now I wish I had those photos to compare—and you will, too! You don't need to share them with anyone else right now if you're self-conscious, but I've had trainees post them on their fridge to remind them of why they were working so hard to get fit. Keep track of your progress with a picture each week; you'll be amazed at your transformation!

Pull-Up

1 Grip the horizontal bar with your palms facing away from you and your arms fully extended. Your hands should be slightly wider (up to 2 inches) than your shoulders. Your feet should not touch the floor during this exercise. Let all of your weight settle in position but don't relax

your shoulders—this may cause them to overstretch.

2 Squeeze your shoulder blades together (scapular retraction) to start the initial phase of the pull-up. During this initial movement, pretend that you're squeezing a pencil between your shoulder blades—don't let the pencil drop during

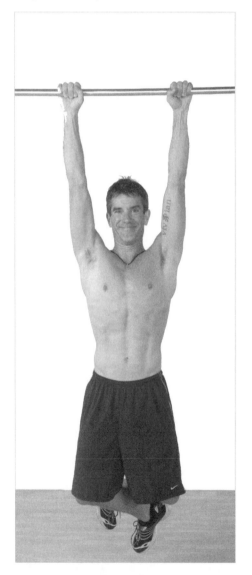

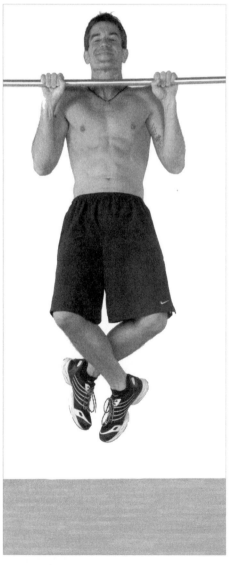

any phase of the pull-up. For phase two (upward/concentric phase), look up at the bar, exhale and pull your chin up toward the bar by driving your elbows toward your hips. It's very important to keep your shoulders back and chest up during the entire movement. Pull yourself up in a controlled manner until the bar is just above the top of your chest.

Inhale and lower yourself back to the starting position.

Be sure to move slowly and with control during both the upward and downward phases. Don't lock your elbows, swing your feet or "bounce" at the bottom of the movement before starting the upward movement. Continue until you've done all the repetitions you can do cleanly.

Write down the number you were able to complete while you take a 2-minute break and prepare for your bodyweight squat test. Whether you complete 0 or 20, make sure to rest the full 2 minutes before moving on to the next exercise.

Squat

1 Stand tall with your feet shoulder-width apart and toes pointed slightly outward, about 11 and 1 o'clock. Raise your arms until they're parallel to the floor.

2 Begin your descent by bending at the hips and "sitting back" just a little bit as if you were about to sit directly down into a chair. Bend your knees slowly and keep your head up, eyes forward and arms out in front of you for balance. Your body should lean forward slightly and your shoulders should almost be in line with your knees; your knees should not extend past your toes. Your weight should remain between the heel and the middle of your feet; don't roll up on the balls of your feet. Stop when your butt is about 6 inches away from the floor or when your knees are at 90° and your thighs are parallel to the floor.

Push straight up from your heels back to the starting position. Don't lock your knees at the top of the exercise. Repeat as many good-form squats as you can.

Write down the number you were able to complete while you take a 2-minute rest and prepare for your push-up test.

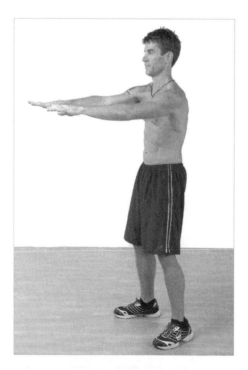
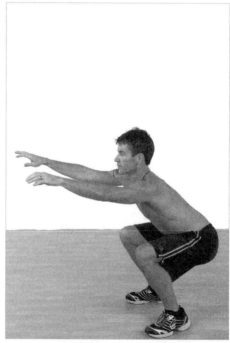

Push-Up

1 Place your hands on the ground approximately shoulder-width apart, making sure your fingers point straight ahead and your arms are straight but your elbows not locked. Step your feet back until your body forms a straight line from head to feet. Your feet should be about 6 inches apart with the weight in the balls of your feet. Engage your core to keep your spine from sagging; don't sink into your shoulders.

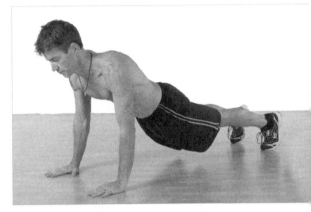

2 Inhale as you lower your torso to the ground and focus on keeping your elbows as close to your sides as possible, stopping when your elbows are at a 90° angle or your chest is 1–2 inches from the floor.

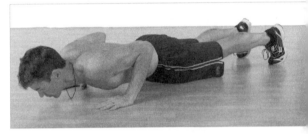

Using your shoulders, chest and triceps, exhale and push your torso back up to starting position. Repeat as many times as you can while using good form.

Write down the number you were able to complete while you take a 2-minute rest and prepare for your final test, the plank.

RIPPED TIP: Sometimes the act of counting your reps can be a mental barrier. Have you ever noticed that when you plan to do 10 repetitions, numbers 8, 9 and 10 are incredibly difficult yet you know you can do 15 reps easily most days? For some people, including me, the act of counting changes the focus on the goal and makes it more difficult to finish. Prior to the exercise, if you think "I never do more than 5," there's a good chance you're mentally limiting yourself before you even start. If you have a partner, have them count your reps inside their head and tell you afterward. Don't have a partner? Use a video camera! Not only can you complete your reps without your mind playing tricks on you, you can also use the footage to check out your form.

Plank

This is a timed exercise, so place a watch where you can see it when you're in position. The plank is exactly like the top portion of a push-up.

THE POSITION: Place your hands on the ground approximately shoulder-width apart, making sure your fingers point straight ahead and your arms are straight but your elbows not locked. Step your feet back until your body forms a straight line from head to feet. Your feet should be about 6 inches apart with the weight in the balls of your feet. Engage your core to keep your spine from sagging; don't sink into your shoulders.

Look at your watch and note the time—you're on the clock. Remember to breathe and maintain the position for as long as you can. Be sure not to let your butt

RIPPED TIP: Engage your core as if you were breathing in and out through a straw—purse your lips and force the air in and out with your ab muscles. Mike DeAngelo would always tell me to "breathe with your belly button" to keep my core taut and back straight.

sag. If you have a partner or mirror, take a peek at your form. Once you can no longer keep your back flat, lower your torso to the floor and note the time.

Congratulations on finishing the test—you're already on your way to getting ripped! Write down your time and grab some water (and maybe even a towel). You're done for today!

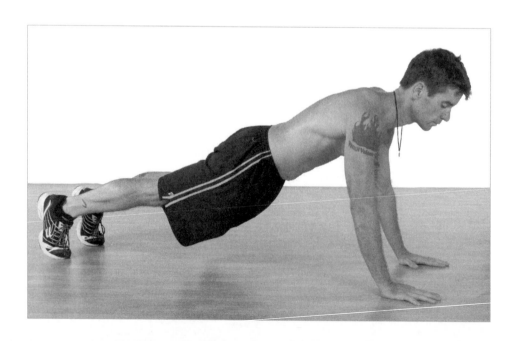

	PULL-UP	PUSH-UP	SQUAT	PLANK
PREP (page 137)	0–5 Reps Completed	0–9 Reps Completed	0–14 Reps Completed	Held for 30 seconds or less
LEVEL I (page 48)	6–11 Reps Completed	10–19 Reps Completed	15–29 Reps Completed	Held for 30–59 seconds
LEVEL II (page 53)	12+	20+	30+	Held for 60–89 seconds

Determining Your Level

Now grab your sheet and let's see how your test performance matches up to the program. Remember, that wasn't a pass/fail test. Any of the different levels will help you get ripped!

Boy, these round numbers are convenient, eh? So, what happens if you're between levels in some areas and not others? Start with the level that has the most reps in common with your initial test. The goal of this book is to get you ripped by working your entire body. You can't do that if you're neglecting any major muscle groups. *Example:* 7 pull-ups, 15 push-ups, 12 squats and a 45-second plank would mean you start with Level I.

Please note: If you were unable to complete any reps on any exercise, it's recommended that you start in the Prep level. For 90 percent of readers, pull-ups will be the deciding factor. It's important that you build them up or you'll be missing a huge part of the program. The Prep level can be found on page 137.

Share Your Success

We've created a Facebook page for our fans to share photos, goals, successes and challenges at facebook.com/7weekstogettingripped. Upload your before, during and after photos to inspire yourself and others. I personally posted my photos during my seven-week transformation and continue to post updates and interact with everyone on the program. Help, tips and motivation are only a click away.

RIPPED TIP: Keep your initial test scores. If you followed an earlier Ripped Tip (see page 37) and took some pictures, print one and write your score on the back. When you complete each program, compare your new test scores with your first score—you should be amazed with your progress.

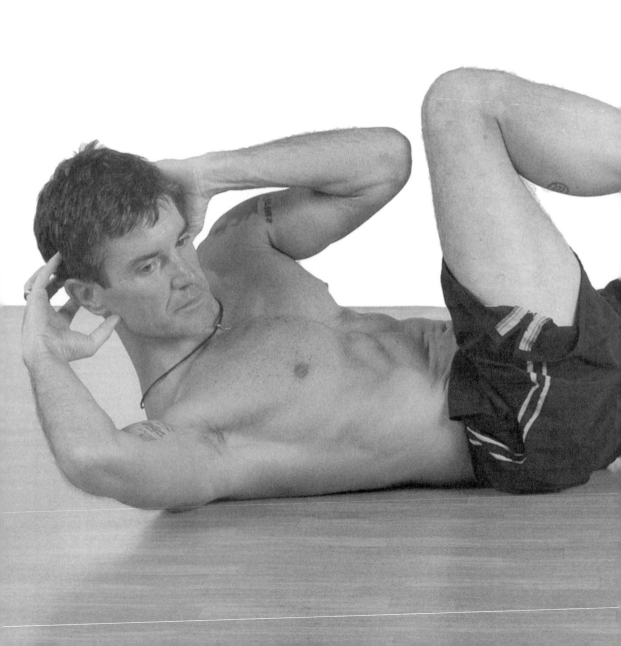

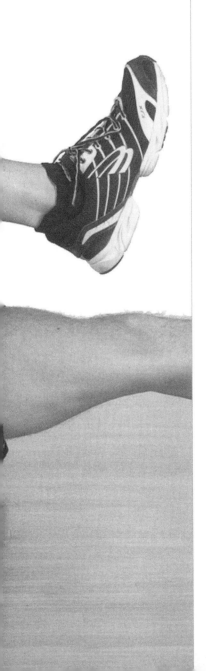

PART II:
THE PROGRAM

7 Weeks to Getting Ripped Program

The *7 Weeks to Getting Ripped* program is composed of two progressive levels (one three weeks long, the other four) and performed three days a week. Each workout is structured around several exercises performed in a superset, with an added cardio component to really kickstart your fat-burning metabolism. *Level I* will build your strength, improve your form and familiarize you with some new exercises that'll help shred your body. *Level II* ratchets up the intensity by adding more complex moves as well as incorporating extreme training methods.

The workouts are performed 3 times a week with at least 1 day of rest in between. From experience, Monday, Wednesday and Friday seem to work the best. If you're planning to start the workout on a Monday, you should take the initial "Power 4" test on the previous Thursday or Friday. If you're new to working out or are returning after some time off, you'll most likely be sore for 1–2 days after taking the initial test. Giving yourself 2–3 days to recover before you start the program is a great idea and increases your chances of success.

Reading the Charts

The program is broken down into a series of weeks. Each week has three "workout" days, so looking at the example for Day 1, Week 1: After warming up for 5 minutes, you'd do 5 chin-ups, 10 squats, 10 push-ups, a 30-second plank and then rest for 2 minutes before starting set 2. Continue

A WORD ABOUT INTENSITY

The higher the level of intensity you put into the workout, the more you'll reap the benefits. Moving from exercise to exercise quickly during supersets, finishing every rep with proper form, putting the hammer down on sprints and speedwork and executing each workout from start to finish is the most efficient way to develop the ripped body you want. The workouts in Level I are challenging, but if you sleepwalk through the movements and slog from one exercise to the next, you're only cheating yourself. Level I is a commitment of about 30 minutes of intense workout 3 days a week. Throw in a game on the weekend and your weekly commitment is only about 2 hours—that's less than some people wait in line per week at their local coffee shop. Stay focused and keep the intensity high throughout your workouts. Don't forget to hydrate and breathe properly, too!

until you've finished all 3 sets and then move on to the cardio/game component before stretching at the end.

Note: Rest and recovery are vital to the success of the programs and should be included as prescribed on the schedules. Remember also to warm up before your workout and stretch afterward! See pages 116–25 for ideas.

Level I

Week 1		Rest 2 minutes after every set (longer if required)			
Mon	*set 1*	5 Chin-Ups	10 Squats	10 Push-Ups	:30 Plank
	set 2	4 Pull-Ups	10 Lunges per leg	9 Narrow Push-Ups	5 V-Sits
	set 3	5 Narrow Chin-Ups	10 Squats	7 Push-Ups	10 In & Outs
	cardio	10 minutes cardio/game			

Level I

Welcome to Level I! By now you've already familiarized yourself with the pull-up, squat, push-up and plank involved in the test, and those will be the "Power 4" exercises that we'll build upon by using different grips, variations and more complex moves. Make no mistake about it—these four simple moves will absolutely shred your body when built into a structured workout that contains variations to mix it up.

Turn to Part III to familiarize yourself with the exercises for each workout before starting. If Day 1 of the workout is too easy for you, please just stick with it for the first week. If you overdo it, you'll miss workouts and it'll be more difficult to get back on track. If you find the workouts still too easy during Week 2, repeat the first set for that day.

Note: Rest and recovery are vital to the success of the programs and should be included as prescribed on the schedules. Remember also to warm up before your workout and stretch afterward! See pages 116–25 for ideas.

Level I

Week 1		Rest 2 minutes after every set (longer if required)			
Mon	set 1	5 Chin-Ups	10 Squats	10 Push-Ups	:30 Plank
	set 2	4 Pull-Ups	10 Lunges per leg	9 Narrow Push-Ups	5 V-Sits
	set 3	5 Narrow Chin-Ups	10 Squats	7 Push-Ups	10 In & Outs
	cardio	10 minutes cardio/game			
Tue		Rest			
Wed	set 1	6 Pull-Ups	12 Squats	10 Push-Ups	:35 Plank
	set 2	5 Chin-Ups	10 Lunges per leg	7 Diamond Push-Ups	16 Supermans
	set 3	5 Narrow Pull-Ups	12 Squats	10 Push-Ups	20 Mason Twists
	cardio	10 minutes cardio/game			
Thu		Rest			
Fri	set 1	6 Chin-Ups	12 Squats	12 Push-Ups	:40 Plank
	set 2	6 Pull-Ups	11 Lunges per leg	10 Narrow Push-Ups	7 Hanging Leg Raises
	set 3	6 Narrow Chin-Ups	12 Squats	12 Push-Ups	10 In & Outs
	cardio	10 minutes cardio/game			
Sat		Rest			
Sun		Rest			

Note: Rest and recovery are vital to the success of the programs and should be included as prescribed on the schedules. Remember also to warm up before your workout and stretch afterward! See pages 116–25 for ideas.

Level I

Week 2		Rest 2 minutes after every set (longer if required)			
Mon	set 1	7 Pull-Ups	12 Squats	12 Push-Ups	:45 Plank
	set 2	7 Chin-Ups	12 Lunges per leg	10 Narrow Push-Ups	7 Supermans
	set 3	7 Narrow Chin-Ups	12 Squats	10 Push-Ups	8 Hanging Leg Raises
	cardio	12 minutes cardio/game			
Tue		Rest			
Wed	set 1	7 Chin-Ups	12 Squats	13 Push-Ups	10 Hanging Leg Raises
	set 2	7 Pull-Ups	10 Wood Chops	10 Push-Ups	20 Mason Twists
	set 3	6 Pull-Ups	12 Lunges per leg	12 Push-Ups	7 V-Sits
	cardio	12 minutes cardio/game			
Thu		Rest			
Fri	set 1	9 Chin-Ups	12 Lunges per leg	12 Push-Ups	12 Hanging Leg Raises
	set 2	8 Pull-Ups	12 Wood Chops	10 Diamond Push-Ups	18 Supermans
	set 3	8 Chin-Ups	14 Squats	10 Push-Ups	:30 Side Plank per side
	cardio	12 minutes cardio/game			
Sat		Rest			
Sun		Rest			

Note: Rest and recovery are vital to the success of the programs and should be included as prescribed on the schedules. Remember also to warm up before your workout and stretch afterward! See pages 116–25 for ideas.

Level I

Week 3		Rest 2 minutes after every set (longer if required)			
Mon	set 1	10 Pull-Ups	15 Squats	14 Push-Ups	14 Hanging Leg Raises
	set 2	11 Chin-Ups	13 Lunges per leg	15 Push-Ups	1:00 Plank
	set 3	8 Pull-Ups	12 Squats	12 Narrow Pull-Ups	24 Mason Twists
	cardio	14 minutes cardio/game			
Tue		Rest			
Wed	set 1	11 Chin-Ups	13 Lunges per leg	15 Push-Ups	1:00 Plank
	set 2	10 Pull-Ups	16 Squats	12 Push-Ups	15 Hanging Leg Raises
	set 3	10 Chin-Ups	12 Lunges per leg	10 Diamond Push-Ups	24 Mason Twists
	cardio	14 minutes cardio/game			
Thu		Rest			
Fri	set 1	10 Pull-Ups	17 Squats	16 Push-Ups	15 Hanging Leg Raises
	set 2	10 Burpees	:30 rest	10 Narrow Push-Ups	1:00 Plank
	set 3	9 Pull-Ups	20 Wood Chops	12 Push-Ups	15 In & Outs
	cardio	14 minutes cardio/game			
Sat		Rest			
Sun		Rest			

Level I Test

Congratulations on completing Level I! You've done some fantastic work to get to this point! Now is a great time to test your progress. Take at least two full days of rest and then take the "Power 4" test again:

- **MAX NUMBER OF PULL-UPS**
(2:00 rest, write down your results)

- **MAX NUMBER OF SQUATS**
(2:00 rest, write down your results)

- **MAX NUMBER OF PUSH-UPS**
(2:00 rest, write down your results)

- **MAX TIME HOLDING A PLANK** (write down your results)

Catch your breath, hydrate and relax. Check your results to see if you should re-take Level I or advance to Level II. How far have you come since your first test? Check out the results on paper—or, better yet, check 'em out in the mirror!

Level II

Congratulations on reaching Level II! This level ratchets up the intensity by adding more complex moves as well as incorporating high-intensity interval training (HIIT) and Tabata intervals.

HIIT is a very effective method for rapid fat burning and performance improvements; it's best described as alternating between maximum intensity for 3–6 reps followed by 3–6 reps at 50% intensity. For sprints, HIIT is maximum effort for a set period of time followed by an equal amount of rest. For example, you'd sprint for 1 minute and then walk for 1 minute, repeating this 8–10 times.

Tabata intervals are extremely short, intense workouts shown to have amazing results in strength building and full-body fat burning. They're based on 20 seconds of superintense exercise followed by 10 seconds of rest. This is repeated for 8 cycles for a total of 3 minutes and 50 seconds. You read that right: less than 4 minutes! Don't underestimate this workout—it'll absolutely exhaust you and help you get shredded like nothing else.

Earlier, we talked a bit about intensity (see page 47) and how important it is to your success with this program. Level II raises the bar with the different intervals and movements featured, but the bottom line is still the same—you'll only get maximum results from the workout if you perform the exercises with good form and at the intensity required for each of the intervals. The goals for Level II are to develop full-body strength and a lean, ripped physique as well as improve your ability to perform all of the movements.

Turn to Part III to familiarize yourself with the exercises for each workout before starting.

Note: Rest and recovery are vital to the success of the programs and should be included as prescribed on the schedules. Remember also to warm up before your workout and stretch afterward! See pages 116–25 for ideas.

Level II

Week 1		Rest 2 minutes after every set (longer if required)					
Mon	set 1	10 Pull-Ups	18 Squats	15 Push-Ups	1:00 Plank	—	—
	set 2	11 Chin-Ups	13 Lunges per leg	14 Narrow Push-Ups	15 Hanging Leg Raises	—	—
	set 3	10 Commando Pull-Ups	10 Squats	12 Diamond Push-Ups	22 Mountain Climbers	—	—
	cardio	15 minutes cardio/game					
Tue		Rest					
Wed	set 1	12 Chin-Ups	10 Lunges with Twist per leg	8 T Push-Ups	14 Air Squats	—	—
	set 2	1:00 Forearm Plank	26 Mountain Climbers	12 Push-Ups	10 Mountain Climbers	12 Supermans	1:00 Forearm Plank
	set 3	10 Pull-Ups	18 Squats	—	—	—	—
	cardio	15 minutes cardio/game					
Thu		Rest					
Fri	set 1	11 Pull-Ups	20 Squats w/Medicine Ball	13 Diamond Push-Ups	18 Hanging Leg Raises	—	—
	set 2	1:10 Plank	10 Burpees	18 Mountain Climbers	30 Wood Chops	—	—
	set 3	15 Chin-Ups	16 Hanging Leg Raises	10 Lunges with Twist per leg	12 Narrow Push-Ups	—	—
	cardio	15 minutes cardio/game					
Sat		Rest					
Sun		Rest					

Note: Rest and recovery are vital to the success of the programs and should be included as prescribed on the schedules. Remember also to warm up before your workout and stretch afterward! See pages 116–25 for ideas.

Level II

Week 2		Rest 2 minutes after every set (longer if required)					
Mon	set 1	12 Pull-Ups	12 Squats	8 T Push-Ups per side	1:15 Plank	—	—
	set 2	12 Chin-Ups	16 Hanging Leg Raises	10 Burpees	8 Push-Ups	—	—
	set 3	10 Pull-Ups	13 Lunges w/ Twist per leg	30 Mountain Climbers	:45 Side Plank per side	12 Supermans	—
	cardio	20 minutes cardio/game					
Tue		Rest					
Wed	set 1	TABATA INTERVALS (10-second rest between reps; repeat 4 times) :20 Squats					
	set 2	TABATA INTERVALS (10-second rest between reps; repeat 4 times) :20 Mountain Climbers					
	set 3	TABATA INTERVALS (10-second rest between each exercise; repeat series 4 times) :20 Jumping Jacks, :20 Butt Kicks; :20 Wood Chops					
	set 4	1:20 Plank					
	cardio	20 minutes cardio/game					
Thu		Rest					
Fri	set 1	14 Pull-Ups	18 Air Squats	13 Diamond Push-Ups	18 Hanging Leg Raises	—	—
	set 2	1:10 Plank	15 T Push-Ups per side	26 Mountain Climbers	30 Wood Chops	—	—
	set 3	15 Chin-Ups	16 Hanging Leg Raises	3 Lunges w/ Twist per leg	10 Burpees	12 Supermans	—
	cardio	20 minutes cardio/game					
Sat		Rest					
Sun		Rest					

Note: Rest and recovery are vital to the success of the programs and should be included as prescribed on the schedules. Remember also to warm up before your workout and stretch afterward! See pages 116–25 for ideas.

Level II

Week 3 — Rest 2 minutes after every set (longer if required)

Mon	set 1	13 Pull-Ups	24 Squats w/Medicine Ball	15 Push-Ups	22 In & Outs	—	—
	set 2	1:20 Plank	15 Narrow Push-Ups	26 Mountain Climbers	30 Wood Chops	—	—
	set 3	15 Chin-Ups	16 Hanging Leg Raises	11 Lunges w/Twist per leg	12 Air Squats	—	—
	cardio	20 minutes cardio/game					
Tue		Rest					
Wed	set 1	12 Chin-Ups	10 Lunges w/Twist per leg	10 Push-Ups	20 Squats	—	—
	set 2	1:00 Forearm Plank	20 Mountain Climbers	5 T Push-Ups per side	20 Reverse Crunches	12 Supermans	:45 Flutter Kicks
	set 3	10 Pull-Ups	24 Wood Chops	—	—	—	—
	cardio	20 minutes cardio/game					
Thu		Rest					
Fri	set 1	12 Commando Pull-Ups	16 Hanging Leg Raises	6 Chin-Ups	8 Hanging Leg Raises	—	—
	set 2	14 Squats	12 Lunges	:30 rest (no further rest between sets)			
	set 3	15 Air Squats	7 Lunges w/Twist per leg	:30 rest (no further rest between sets)			
	set 4	1:00 Plank	26 Mountain Climbers	12 Medicine Ball Push-Ups	—	—	—
	cardio	20 minutes cardio/game					
Sat		Rest					
Sun		Rest					

Note: Rest and recovery are vital to the success of the programs and should be included as prescribed on the schedules. Remember also to warm up before your workout and stretch afterward! See pages 116–25 for ideas.

Level II

Week 4		Rest 2 minutes after every set (longer if required)				
Mon	*set 1*	TABATA INTERVALS (10-second rest between reps; repeat 4 times) :20 Air Squats				
	set 2	TABATA INTERVALS (10-second rest between reps; repeat 4 times) :20 Mountain Climbers				
	set 3	TABATA INTERVALS (10-second rest between each exercise; repeat series 4 times) :20 Jumping Jacks; :20 Butt Kicks; :20 Wood Chops				
	set 4	1:20 Plank	1:00 rest (no further rest between sets)			
	cardio	20 minutes cardio/game				
Tue		Rest				
Wed	*set 1*	14 Pull-Ups	26 Squats w/Medicine Ball	18 Push-Ups	1:15 Plank	—	—
	set 2	15 Commando Pull-Ups	16 Hanging Leg Raises	30 Wood Chops	12 Medicine Ball Push-Ups	—	—
	set 3	14 Burpees	13 Lunges w/ Twist per leg	30 Mountain Climbers	:45 Flutter Kicks	12 Supermans	—
	cardio	20 minutes cardio/game				
Thu		Rest				
Fri	*set 1*	20 Squats w/Medicine Ball	6 Lunges w/ Twist per leg	:30 rest (no further rest between sets)		
	set 2	12 Pull-Ups	16 Hanging Leg Raises	5 Pull-Ups	10 Hanging Leg Raises	—	—
	set 3	15 Air Squats	7 Lunges w/ Twist per leg	:30 rest (no further rest between sets)		
	set 4	1:00 Plank	30 Mountain Climbers	12 Medicine Ball Push-Ups	12 Supermans	—	—
	cardio	20 minutes cardio/game				
Sat		Rest				
Sun		Rest				

Level II Test

Congratulations on completing Level II! I hope you've gotten a whole bunch of amazing workouts under your belt and learned some great new moves! What do you think, is this a good time to test your progress? Sure, why not? Take at least two full days of rest and then take the "Power 4" test again:

- **MAX NUMBER OF PULL-UPS**
  (2:00 rest, write down your results)

- **MAX NUMBER OF SQUATS**
  (2:00 rest, write down your results)

- **MAX NUMBER OF PUSH-UPS**
  (2:00 rest, write down your results)

- **MAX TIME HOLDING A PLANK** (write down your results)

Catch your breath, hydrate and relax. How far have you come since your first test?

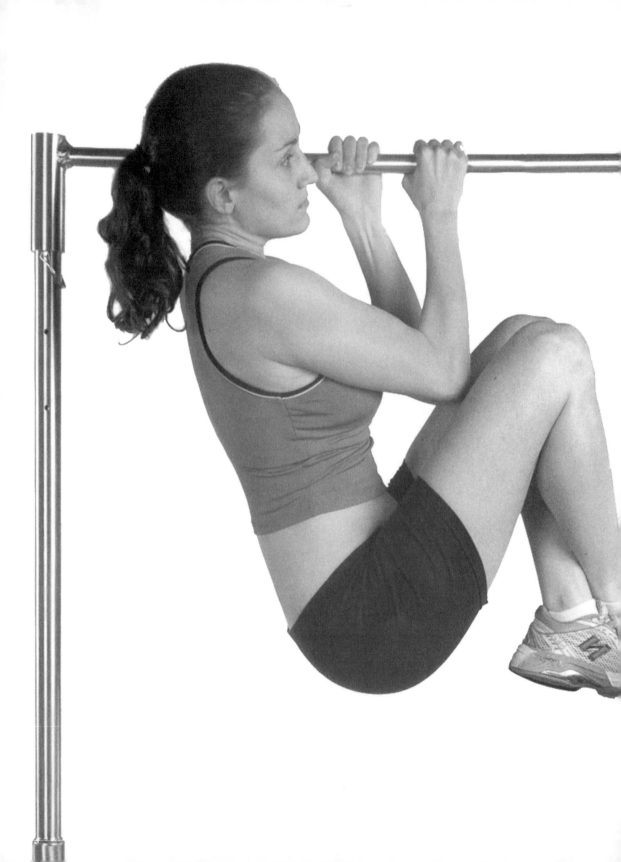

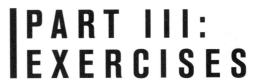

PART III:
EXERCISES

Standard Push-Up

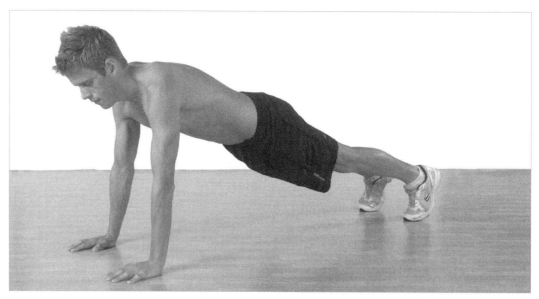

1 Place your hands on the ground approximately shoulder-width apart, making sure your fingers point straight ahead and your arms are straight but your elbows not locked. Step your feet back until your body forms a straight line from head to feet. Your feet should be about 6 inches apart with the weight in the balls of your feet. Engage your core to keep your spine from sagging; don't sink into your shoulders.

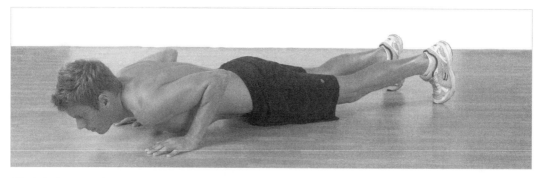

2 Inhale as you lower your torso to the ground and focus on keeping your elbows as close to your sides as possible, stopping when your elbows are at a 90° angle or your chest is 1–2 inches from the floor.

Using your shoulders, chest and triceps, exhale and push your torso back up to starting position.

STAGGERED VARIATION: Staggered push-ups can be done with your hands in pretty much any position as long as you can support yourself. Be aware of any pain in your elbows or shoulders; moving your hands away from your torso increases the load these joints need to bear to lower and raise your body.

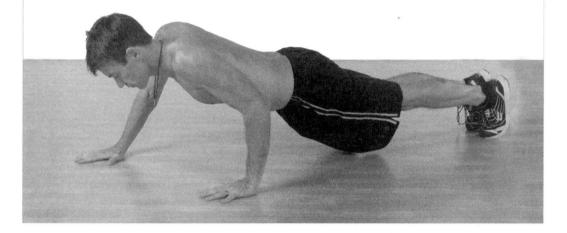

Diamond Push-Up

This version targets the triceps more than standard push-ups do.

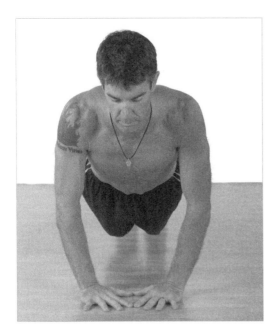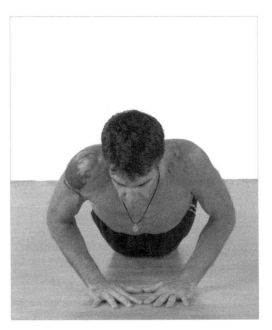

Place your hands directly under your chest with the thumb and forefinger of each hand touching to form a "diamond."

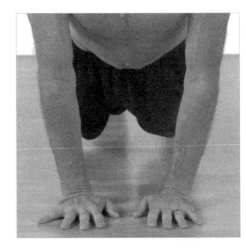

NARROW VARIATION: This version also targets the triceps more than standard push-ups do. Here, your hands are 6–10 inches apart.

Wide Push-Up

This move does a good job of isolating your chest.

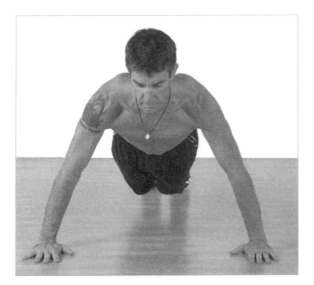

Place your hands anywhere from 6 to 12 inches away from your chest on either side. Be aware of any pain in your elbows or shoulders; moving your hands away from your torso increases the load these joints need to bear to lower and raise your body.

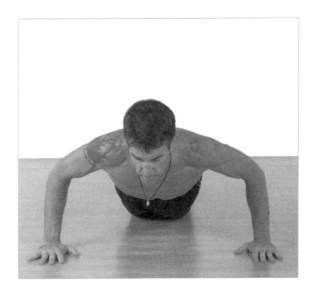

Medicine Ball Push-Up

Medicine ball push-ups require you to use a host of different supporting muscles throughout your upper body and core to stay stable while you complete the movement.

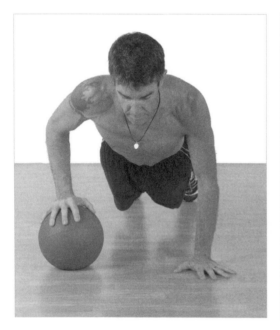

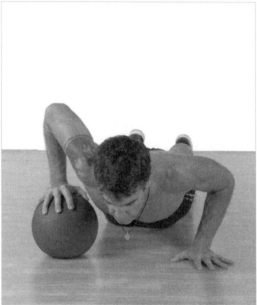

1 Assume a push-up position but place a medicine ball under one hand while keeping the other hand flat on the floor. Engage your core to keep your spine erect and keep your body in a straight line from head to toe.

2 Inhale as you lower your upper body toward the floor, stopping when your chest is about 1 inch above the medicine ball.

Exhale and push off the floor using your arms, chest, back and core and return to starting position.

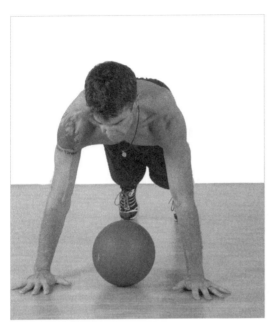

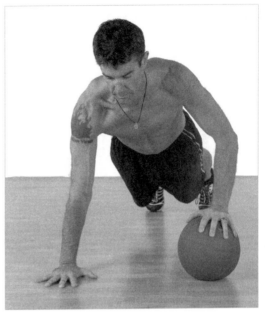

3–4 Place both hands on the floor and walk your hands to the left or right to place your other hand on top of the ball. Repeat until all reps are complete.

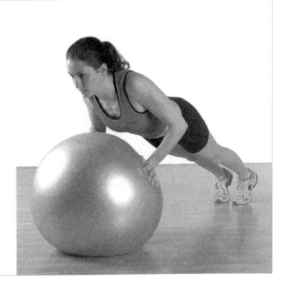

VARIATION: With larger medicine balls or stability balls, you can work your supporting muscles even more by placing both hands on one ball and performing a push-up. Perform the push-up with careful attention to keeping your core taut and maintaining your balance. A good grip is extremely important, so be careful using any ball with a slippery surface.

T Push-Up

This exercise gets its name from the ending position when your body forms a "T."

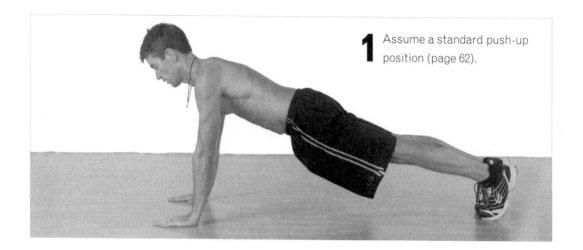

1 Assume a standard push-up position (page 62).

2 Inhale as you lower your torso to the ground, stopping when your elbows are at a 90° angle or your chest is 1–2 inches from the floor.

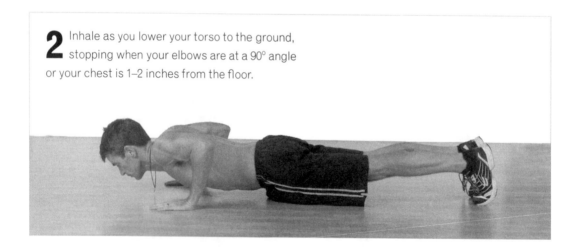

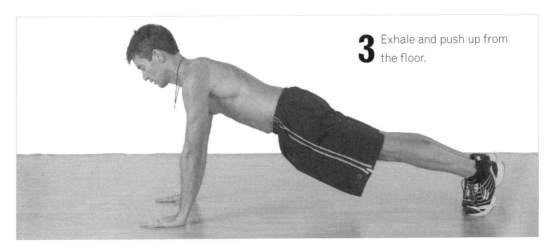

3 Exhale and push up from the floor.

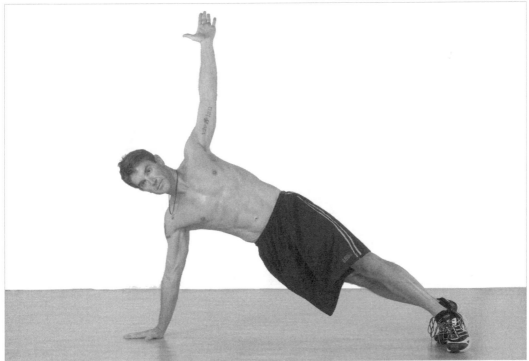

4 As your arms near full extension, lift your left hand off the floor and slowly raise your hand out to your left side while simultaneously rotating your entire torso, head and left leg until your body forms a "T" shape with your left arm pointing directly upward and your right hand in contact with the floor, supporting your weight. Maintain a contracted core and keep your spine erect. Hold that position for 3 seconds (or longer if you choose to incorporate a side plank).

Slowly rotate your torso back to plank position. Repeat on the other side.

Pull-Up

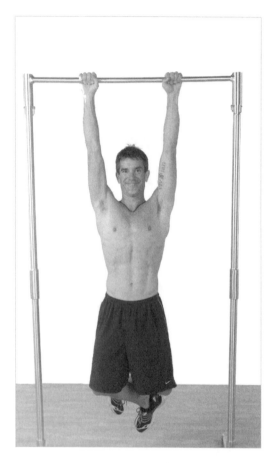 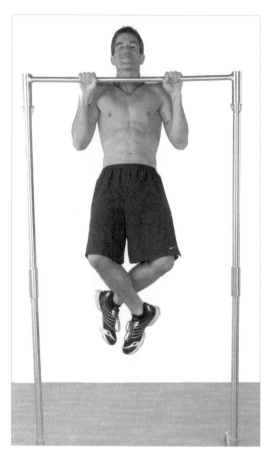

1 Grip the horizontal bar with your palms facing away from you and your arms fully extended. Your hands should be slightly wider (up to 2 inches) than your shoulders. Your feet should not touch the floor during this exercise. Let all of your weight settle in position but don't relax your shoulders—this may cause them to overstretch.

2 Squeeze your shoulder blades together (scapular retraction) to start the initial phase of the pull-up. During this initial movement, pretend that you're squeezing a pencil between your shoulder blades—don't let the pencil drop during any phase of the pull-up. For phase two (upward/concentric phase), look up at the bar, exhale and pull your chin up toward the bar by driving your elbows toward your hips. It's very important to keep your shoulders back and chest up during the entire movement. Pull yourself up in a controlled manner until the bar is just above the top of your chest.

Inhale and lower yourself back to starting position.

Pull-Up Grip Variations

While the overall pull-up movement and muscles activated are the same, each grip variation has its own advantages, targeting slightly different muscles. It's a great idea to rotate through different grips during each set of pull-up exercises. Here are the main recommended grips listed from easiest to hardest:

UNDERHAND (CHIN-UP) GRIP: Grab the bar with your palms facing you. This movement is easiest because it allows you to use more of your biceps to complete the motion. On average, underhand pull-ups are about 10–15 percent easier than overhand pull-ups.

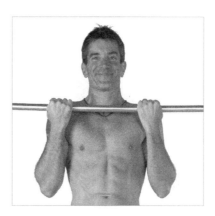

NARROW GRIP: Grab the bar (underhand or overhand) with your hands 3–6 inches apart. Because of the close proximity of your hands, you may need to lean back a bit so you don't smack your face on the backs of your hands. Also, due to the compact nature of bringing your arms in medially, you'll engage your core a bit more than during a standard overhand pull-up. Narrow-grip overhand pull-ups are generally easier than a standard overhand pull-up and emphasize the lower lats.

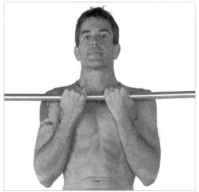

NEUTRAL GRIP: In order to do this type of pull-up, you'll need to use a pull-up apparatus with handles that are 90° in relation to a normal pull-up bar. These handles will allow you to create a hand position where your palms are facing each other about 8–12 inches apart. Neutral pull-ups are the most natural hand position and allow significant use of the biceps, upper chest and core. With neutral pull-ups, it's important to remember to engage your upper back muscles, as it's possible to "cheat" and use your biceps as the prime movers.

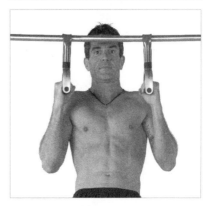

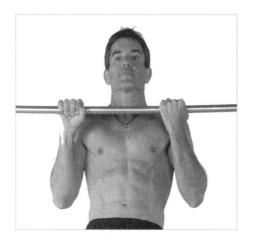

MIXED GRIP: This is done with one overhand grip and one underhand grip. Due to the imbalances caused by mixing your grip, you'll work more core and upper-body stabilizing muscles than you would with either the underhand or overhand grips. Since most people will use the biceps of the underhand-grip arm to do more than its fair share of work to complete the move, you should swap grips in-between sets if you're doing multiples or split the set in half and swap in the middle.

WIDE GRIP: The wide-grip pull-up, with hands on the bar about 8–12 inches outside the shoulders, is an advanced move and should only be performed by well-trained, fit individuals. Often, pull-up bars will have a 45° bend near the ends; this is where you should place your hands if your arms are long enough. The angle of the bar is more anatomically correct and easier on your shoulders. This is the hardest pull-up hand position for a few reasons. Mainly, moving

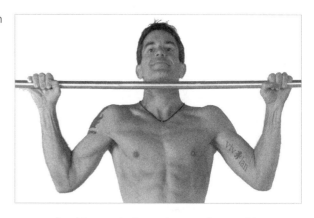

your hands laterally away from your core places your shoulders and elbows in a weaker position. Stabilizer muscles that normally aren't responsible for carrying a large amount of weight are now really "on the hook" to assist your arms and latissimus dorsi. This effectively increases your overall upper back strength, but with a caveat—the strain put on your rotator cuffs and elbows may cause pain or even joint failure. Used sparingly, it's a good test of your overall upper back strength, but please stop at the first sign of any elbow or shoulder pain.

Commando Pull-Up

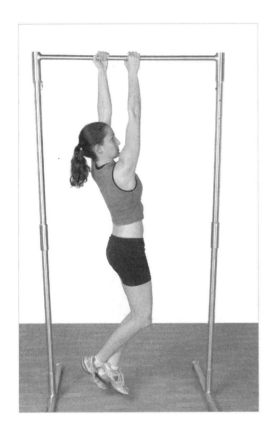 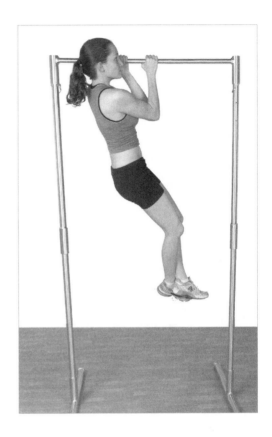

1 Stand perpendicular to the bar with it directly overhead and bisecting your body into left and right halves. Reach up to grip the bar like a baseball bat (e.g., hands on opposite sides of the bar). Your elbows should be a few inches apart and pointed toward the floor, not flared out to the sides.

2 Engage your core and pull upward using your biceps, shoulder, chest and back to bring your head up on one side of the bar. Keep your arms tight to your torso and bring your elbows toward your waist. At the top of the move, touch one shoulder to the bar.

In a slow and controlled manner, lower your body back to the starting position. Switch shoulders each rep.

RIPPED VARIATION: For more core activation, on the upward movement raise your knees up and crunch your core—the higher your legs, the more you activate your core. You can even bring your feet up to touch the bar.

Plank

This is a timed exercise, so place a watch where you can see it when you're in position.

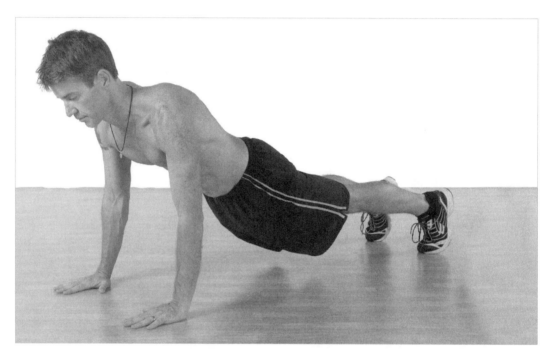

1 Place your hands on the ground approximately shoulder-width apart, making sure your fingers point straight ahead and your arms are straight but your elbows not locked. Step your feet back until your body forms a straight line from head to feet. Your feet should be about 6 inches apart with the weight in the balls of your feet. Engage your core to keep your spine from sagging; don't sink into your shoulders. Look at your watch and note the time—you're on the clock.

Lower to starting position when time is reached.

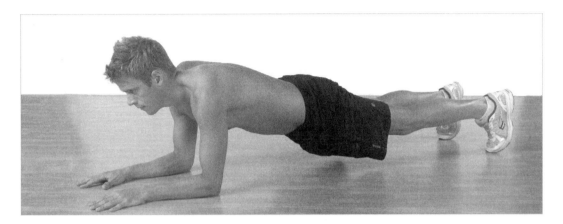

FOREARM VARIATION: Place your elbows on the floor beneath your shoulders, your hands palm-down on the floor and your entire forearms in contact with the floor. Because your body is closer to parallel with the floor, you're working your core even harder to maintain a straight line from head to toe.

CHECKING YOUR LINE

Use a training partner, mirror or even a straight object like a broom handle to make sure your body is straight (you'll have a little curve at the bottom of your spine above the pelvis—that's normal). If you have a four-foot piece of PVC pipe, you can make your planks superchallenging and fun: Get into forearm plank position (it works best when you're closer to parallel with the floor) and have a partner place the PVC pipe on your back, resting it between your shoulder blades, down your spine and across your buttocks. Time each other to see who can keep the pipe from rolling off the longest. If you want to kick it up a notch, you can put some sand in the PVC pipe and cap the ends for weighted planks.

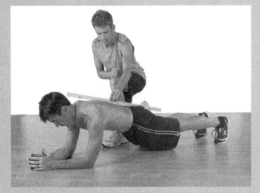

Side Plank

The side plank is a great isolation exercise for tightening your internal and external abdominal obliques (aka your love handles) as well as the transverse abdominis. For some people with lower back problems that prevent them from twisting with a full range of motion, side plank may be a beneficial exercise, but it's not perfect for all. The instability of the side plank will work a host of supporting muscles all over your body, including your hips, glutes, chest and back. On average, side planks are held for about half as long as standard planks.

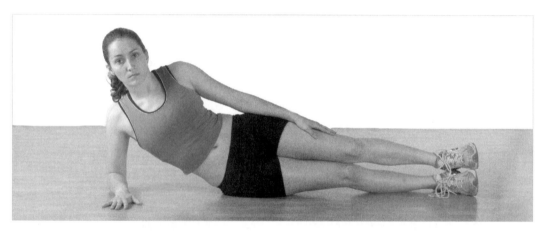

1 Lie on your side and stack your feet, hips and shoulders atop each other. Prop yourself up on your elbow, keeping it directly under your shoulder; your forearm should be completely on the ground, perpendicular to your body.

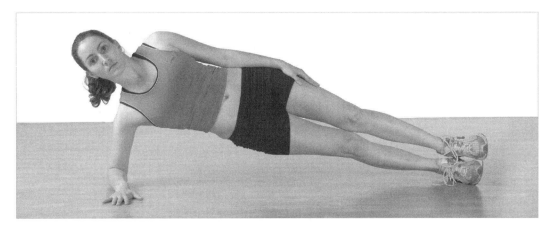

2 Engaging your core to keep your spine erect, lift your hips off the floor until you form a nice line from head to feet. Let your top arm rest along your side. Hold the position for a predetermined amount of time or for as long as possible.

Slowly lower your hips to the floor. Repeat on the opposite side.

MODIFICATION: People with weak knees may find that this position puts a great deal of strain on their knees when they keep both legs straight. To alleviate some of the stress, I've used a foam roller, medicine ball or similar to provide some knee joint stability. Place the object on the outside of the thigh that is closest to the ground and keep your legs straight. You may need to experiment with the positioning to get comfortable.

In & Out

Aside from planks, this is my favorite core move due to its full range of motion and how well it works the entire rectus abdominis and erector spinae without putting excessive force on your upper spine and neck. Because your hands are not placed behind your neck like an old-school sit-up, there's no tendency to jerk your head forward; the transverse lateral arm motion helps to keep your shoulders level and encourages you to complete the movement. We're all fans of immediate feedback and you know right away if you're cheating if your arms are not level to the floor. This is a very slow and controlled motion and is performed best at a cadence of 3 seconds in, 3 seconds hold and 3 seconds out.

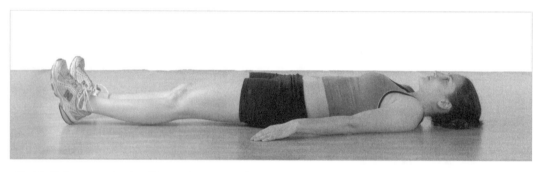

1 Lie flat on your back with your legs extended straight along the floor and your arms along your sides, palms down.

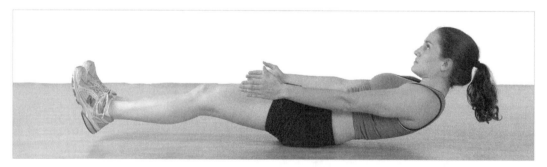

2 Lift your feet about 3 inches off the floor, bend your knees and bring your feet toward your butt while simultaneously lifting your arms off the floor and activating your abs to roll your upper body upward.

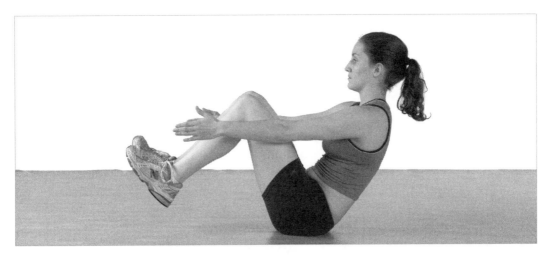

3 Continue raising your head and shoulders off the floor and bringing your hands past the outside of your knees while bringing your knees and chest together. At the top of the move, pause for 1–3 seconds.

Slowly return to starting position. Be careful to "roll" your spine in a natural movement and let your shoulders and head lightly touch the floor.

VARIATION: For more abs activation, maintain the same distance of your feet from the floor as you extend your legs back to straight and hold them there until you begin the next rep. It's a lot harder and you'll recruit far more muscles from your upper legs, pelvic girdle and hips to extend your legs in and out without letting your heels touch. Remember to keep your hands level to the floor—you're cheating if you raise them up!

Flutter Kick

My high school gym teacher used to call these "6 inches."

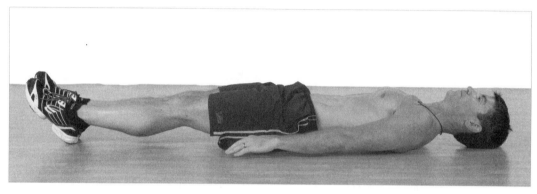

1 Lie flat on your back with your legs extended along the floor and your arms along your sides, palms down.

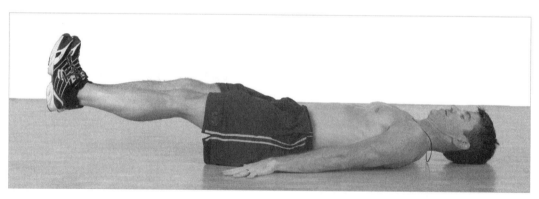

2 Contract your lower abdominal muscles and lift your feet 6 inches off the floor. Hold for 5 seconds. (I prefer to flex my feet 90° in order to work my calves a bit, but you may point your toes.)

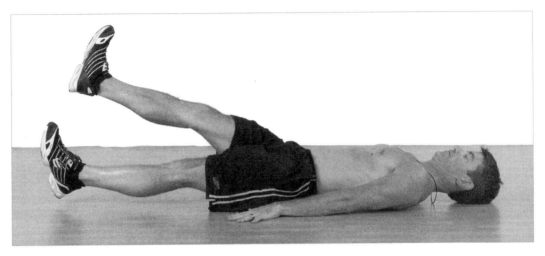

3 While keeping your left foot in place, lift your right foot 6 inches higher (it should now be 12 inches off the floor). Hold for 5 seconds.

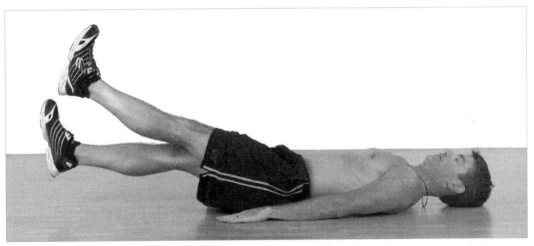

4 Simultaneously lower your right leg back to 6 inches off the floor while raising your left foot 6 inches higher. Hold for 5 seconds.

This counts as 2 reps.

Mason Twist

This exercise works the oblique abdominal muscles, the erector spinae and even the hip flexors. Always be careful when using weights in a twisting motion as you can easily injure your lower back. Start with the lightest possible weight and work your way up as you become more comfortable with the move and refine your form.

1 Sit on the floor with your knees comfortably bent, feet on the floor, arms bent 90° and hands holding a medicine ball or weight in front of your chest.

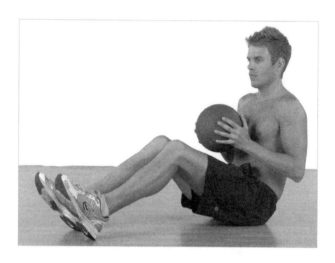

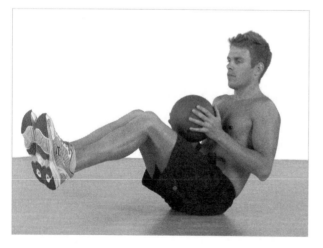

2 Lift your feet 4–6 inches off the floor and balance your bodyweight on your posterior. Keep your core tight to protect your back.

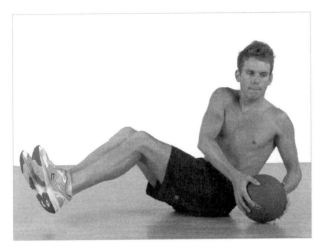

3 While maintaining the same hip position, twist your entire torso at the waist and touch the ball to the floor on the left side of your body.

4 Rotate back to center, keeping your feet off the floor and maintaining your balance using the supporting core muscles. Then rotate to your right and touch the ball to the floor.

Return to center. This is one rep.

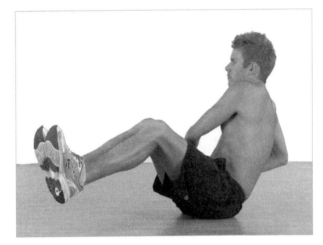

MODIFICATION: If you're not ready to add weight, you can also do this by clasping your hands in front of you.

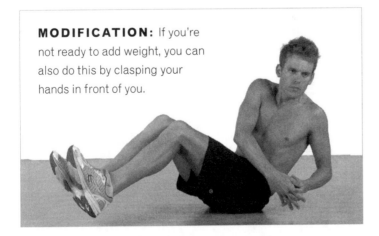

V-Sit

This is one of those exercises that sounds exactly how it looks but, boy, is it tougher than it sounds. This is a slow, controlled movement: Never jerk your body from a prone dorsal position to a V—that's a quick way to pull a muscle! In order to reap the benefits of this exercise and the host of supporting muscles it works (not to mention the coordination it helps build), really focus on your form and practice keeping your core engaged and mirroring the straightness of your upper body and legs. It also doesn't hurt to have a soft cushion under your tailbone.

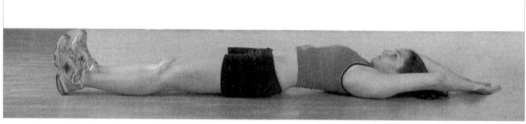

1 Lie flat on your back with your legs extended straight along the floor and your arms extended overhead on the floor with your biceps by your ears.

2 Contracting your abdominal muscles and keeping your legs straight, raise your legs and upper torso to form a "V." Your straight arms can be held parallel to your legs or alongside your ears. Hold the position for at least 3 seconds.

Slowly lower everything down without touching the ground with your heels or shoulders, then perform another rep.

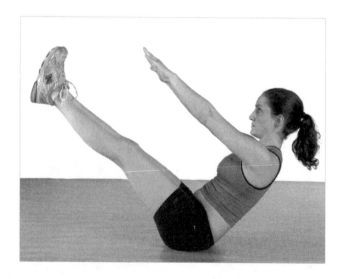

Reverse Crunch

Keep your back straight and lower legs on a level plane throughout this slow and controlled movement.

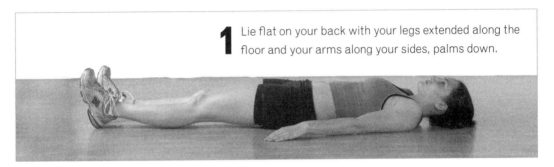

1 Lie flat on your back with your legs extended along the floor and your arms along your sides, palms down.

2 Contracting your lower abdominal muscles, lift your feet 4–6 inches off the floor, bend your knees and bring them in toward your chest. Be careful not to put excessive pressure on your lower back by bringing your hips off the floor. Pause when your glutes rise slightly off the mat.

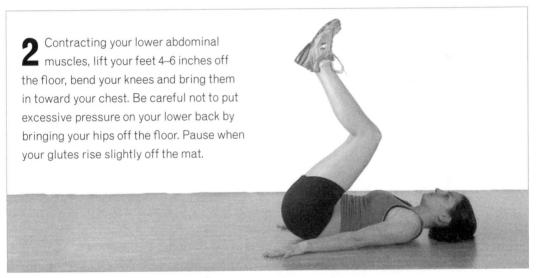

3 Extend your legs and lower them until your feet are 4–6 inches off the floor.

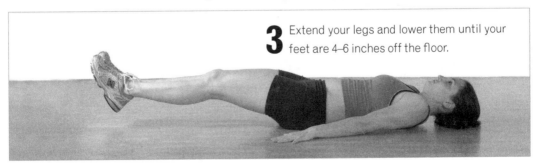

Hanging Leg Raise

This is a great movement to work your lower abdominal muscles and hips while also providing a great stretch for your arms, shoulders and back. Don't be surprised if your vertebrae re-align themselves when you first hang and even throughout the move; this is one of those rare times in life when there are no impactful forces on your spine, so enjoy it.

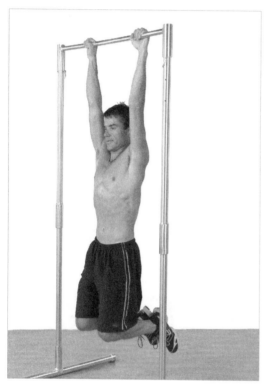 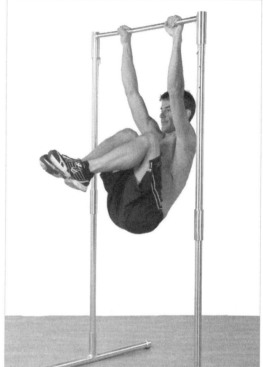

1 Grab an overhead bar with your preferred grip (underhand, overhand or mixed) and hang from the bar with your arms fully extended but elbows not locked. For this exercise, count 3 seconds up, hold 1–3 seconds, and then 3 seconds down.

2 Contracting your abdominal muscles, slowly bring your knees up toward your chest while keeping your torso as close to vertical as possible. Don't lean back during the movement or swing between reps.

Lower your legs in the same slow manner.

RIPPED VARIATION: Kick your hanging leg raises up a notch by adding a pike on the way down. After you bring your legs to your chest and hold for 3 seconds, straighten your legs as you lower them and hold in a pike position (or "L" shape formed by your torso and legs) for an additional 3 seconds. Ready for more? Hold the pike position and do some pull-ups.

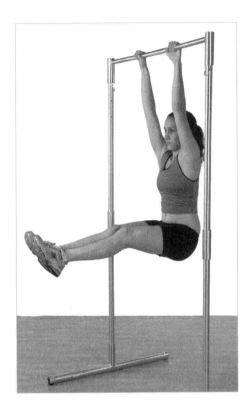

Leg Climber

This move could best be described as a one-legged V-sit (page 84), but incorporates some obliques by twisting to grab one leg and literally climb your hands up it. This slow, controlled movement takes some time to master and even longer to look good while doing it.

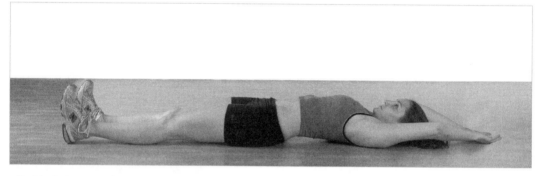

1 Lie flat on your back with your legs extended straight along the floor and your arms extended overhead on the floor with your biceps by your ears.

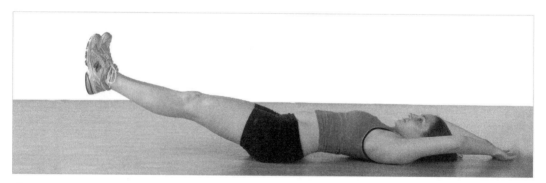

2 Contract your abdominal muscles and raise both legs off the ground 8–12 inches. Keep both legs straight.

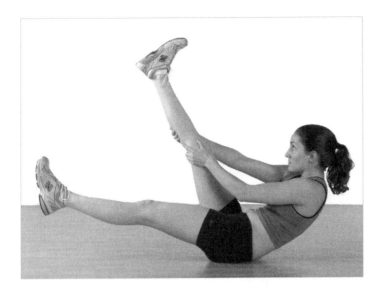

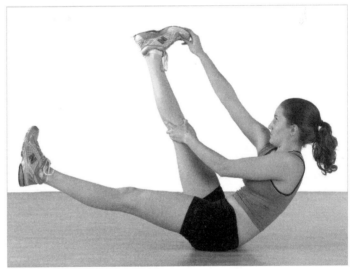

3–4 Keeping your left leg in place, raise your right leg and your upper torso very similar to the V-sit. Reach your left hand to grab the inside of your right leg (the higher the better), then grab the same leg closer to your foot with your right hand. Work your hands up until you've successfully climbed Mount (insert your name here)'s leg. If done properly, you should look a little like someone trying to examine their right toenails in the least effective manner—right foot in hand, torso and right leg in a V and left leg sticking out trying to maintain balance.

Bicycle Crunch

1 Lie flat on your back with your legs extended straight along the floor and your hands at both sides of your head, fingers touching your temples.

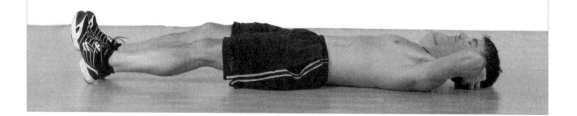

2 Raise your feet 6 inches off the floor while simultaneously contracting your rectus abdominis and lifting your upper back and shoulders off the floor. In one movement, bend your left knee and raise your left leg so that the thigh and shin are at 90°; rotate your torso using your oblique muscles so that your right elbow touches the inside of your left knee.

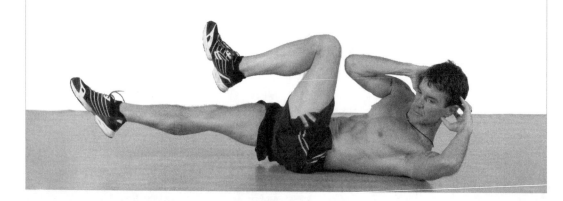

3 Rotate your torso back to center and lower your upper body toward the floor, stopping before your shoulders touch.

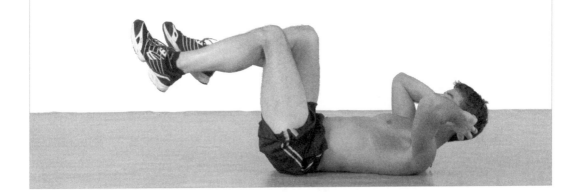

4 Extend your left knee and return your foot to 6 inches off the floor and bend your right leg to 90°. Contract your abs, rotate and touch your left elbow to the inside of your right knee. This is 2 reps.

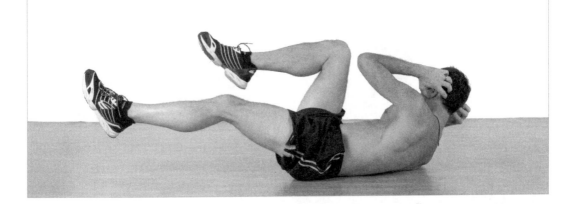

Superman

Interestingly enough, this exercise is not performed "up, up and away" but actually on your stomach, flat on the ground. However, the Man of Steel would greatly appreciate the importance of this move as it strengthens your lower back and gives some due attention to your erector spinae—you know, those muscles that keep you vertical.

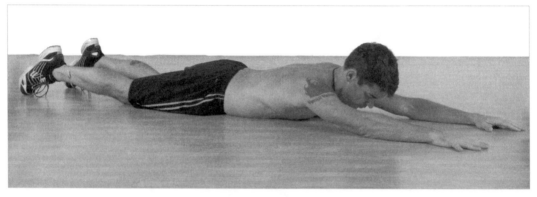

1 Lying face down on your stomach, extend your arms directly out in front of you and your legs behind you. Keep your knees straight as if you were flying.

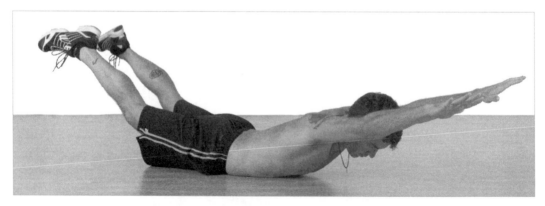

2 In a slow and controlled manner, contract your erector spinae and raise your arms and legs about 6–8 inches off the floor. Hold for 5 seconds.

Lower slowly back to starting position.

Squat

Squat form is crucial to getting the most out of this extremely beneficial exercise. Check out your form by using a full-body mirror and standing perpendicular to it as you complete your reps.

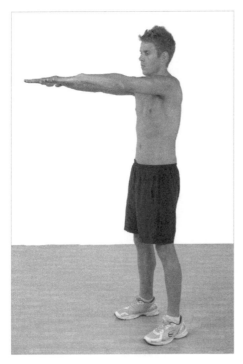

1 Stand tall with your feet shoulder-width apart and toes pointed slightly outward, about 11 and 1 o'clock. Raise your arms until they're parallel to the floor.

2 Bend at the hips and knees and "sit back" just a little bit as if you were about to sit directly down into a chair. Keep your head up, eyes forward and arms out in front of you for balance. As you descend, contract your glutes while your body leans forward slightly so that your shoulders are almost in line with your knees. Your knees should not extend past your toes and your weight should remain between the heel and the middle of your feet—do not roll up on the balls of your feet. Stop when your knees are at 90° and your thighs are parallel to the floor. If you feel your weight is on your toes or heels, adjust your posture and balance until your weight is in the middle of your feet. Squats should be a very stable movement—that is, until you try the one-legged variety!

Push straight up from your heels back to starting position. Don't lock your knees at the top of the exercise. This is 1 rep.

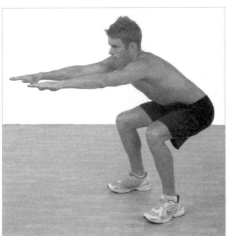

AIR SQUAT VARIATION: For this version, lower yourself into a squat position then swing your arms up and explode straight up in the air. Land softly on your feet.

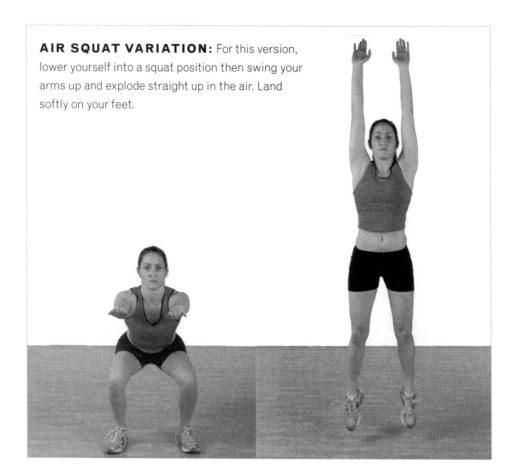

Squat with Medicine Ball

The medicine ball provides some additional weight to the squat and also works your arms, core and a litany of connecting muscles by changing your point of balance throughout the move. As an added benefit, it gives you something useful to do with your hands.

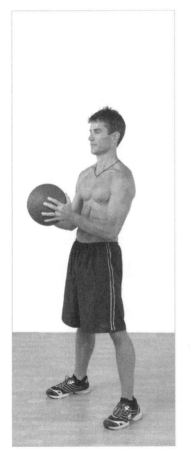 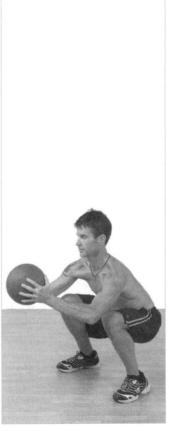 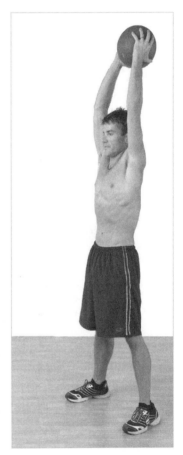

1 Stand tall with your feet shoulder-width apart and toes pointed slightly outward, about 11 and 1 o'clock. Hold a medicine ball at chest level.

2 Keeping the ball in front of you, perform a traditional squat. When your knees near 90°, stop and slowly return to standing.

3 Exhale and raise the ball straight up overhead.

Slowly lower the ball back to chest level.

Wall Sit

While this motion is very similar to a squat, wall sits are a timed exercise much akin to a plank (page 74). The goal is to increase your leg strength. This move is actually tougher than it seems and a good exercise to mix in with squats and lunges if you get bored.

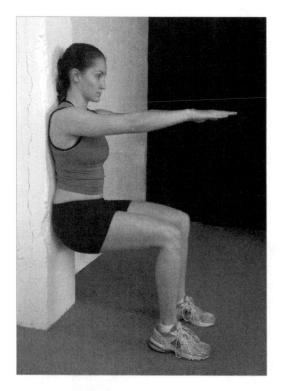
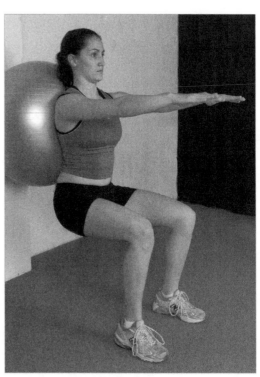

THE POSITION: Place your back flat against a stable wall and walk your feet out, sliding your back down the wall, until your upper and lower legs are at a 90° angle. Keeping your head up, core engaged and spine straight, breathe normally as you begin to count. You can place your hands on your knees if you need extra support, let them hang by your sides, or raise them overhead or straight out.

BALL VARIATION: Place a stability ball between your back and the wall and perform a traditional wall sit. This really works a ton of connecting muscles in your lower body and core.

Forward Lunge

1 Stand tall with your feet shoulder-width apart and your arms hanging at your sides.

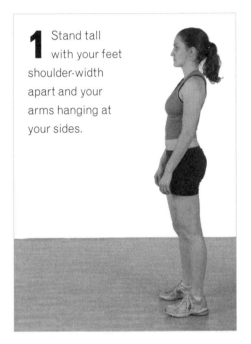

2 Take a large step forward with your right foot, bend both knees and drop your hips straight down until both knees are bent 90°. Your left knee should almost be touching the ground and your left toes are on the ground behind you. Keep your core engaged and your back, neck and hips straight at all times during this movement.

Pushing up with your right leg, straighten both knees and return to starting position. Repeat with the other leg.

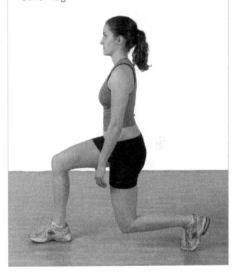

REVERSE VARIATION: Reverse lunges are just like their forward counterparts, but begin by taking a step backward. These can be slightly more difficult to maintain your balance and are a bit better for activating supporting muscles in your pelvis, legs and core.

Lunge with Twist

This movement is exactly like the forward or reverse lunge, but now your hands and core can get in on the fun.

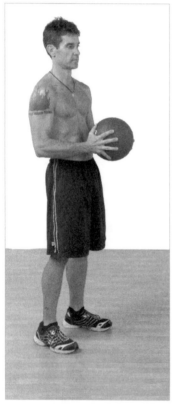 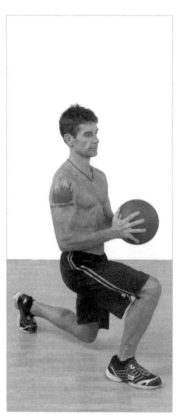 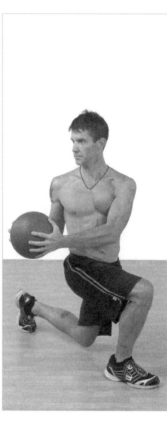

1 Stand tall with your feet shoulder-width apart and both hands on opposite sides of a medicine ball, elbows slightly bent.

2–3 Keeping the ball directly in front of you, step forward (or backward) with your right foot to start the lunge motion. As you lower your hips, twist your core and swing the ball laterally to your right until both knees are bent 90° and your arms are extended and holding the medicine ball to the right, 90° from where you started.

Return to starting position and repeat to the other side.

Marching Twist

Start slowly and work up the intensity. You can even throw in some intervals to really raise your heart rate.

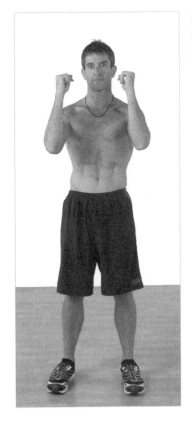 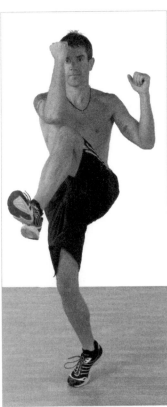 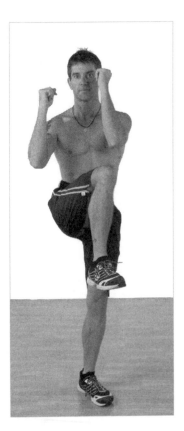

1 Stand tall with your feet shoulder-width apart. Bring your arms in front of you and bend your elbows 90°.

2 Twist your torso to the left and raise your left knee to your right elbow.

3 Repeat with your right knee and left elbow. A little hop with the bottom foot helps you keep your momentum going from leg to leg.

Mountain Climbers

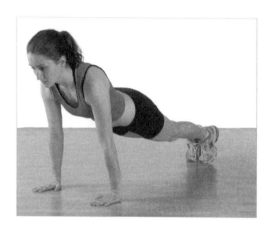

1 Assume the top position of a push-up with your hands directly under your shoulders and toes on the ground. Keep your core engaged and your body in a straight line from head to toe.

2 Lift your right toe slightly off the ground, bring your right knee to your chest and place your right foot on the ground under your body.

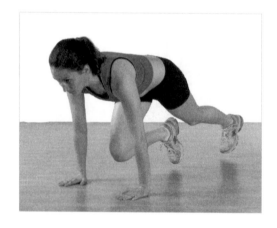

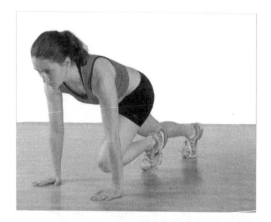

3 With a very small hop from both toes, extend your right foot back to starting position and at the same time bring your left knee to your chest and place your left foot on the ground under your body.

Continue switching, making sure to keep your hips low.

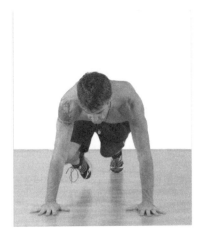 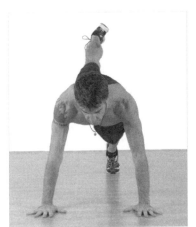

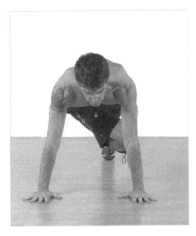 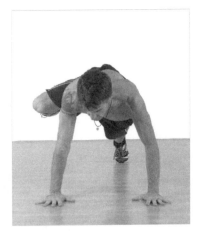

ADVANCED VARIATION: This advanced move really works the core (it's essentially a plank with a lot of leg movement) and strengthens your glutes and hips. Instead of hopping and switching your legs, you'll bring your right knee toward your right shoulder and then extend it straight out behind you (this is the "mule kick," so lift your foot as high as possible while keeping your hips firmly in place; do not rock or raise your butt!). Without touching your foot to the ground, bring your right knee toward your left shoulder before extending it for another mule kick. Lastly, raise your leg laterally (picture a male dog around a fire hydrant) and bring your knee toward your right shoulder, then finish the move with yet another mule kick before returning your right foot back to starting position. Now repeat with your left leg.

Burpee

The burpee combines a squat, a double-leg mountain climber, a push-up and a high jump. It's a great full-body workout that you can do anywhere to work up a sweat and target your arms, chest, glutes, quads, hamstrings, calves and core. Since it's a multiple-position movement, take the time to learn and practice proper position for each move before you try it at full speed.

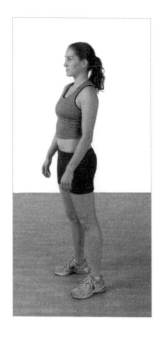

1 Stand tall with your back erect, feet shoulder-width apart and toes rotated slightly outward.

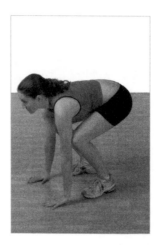

2 Shift your hips backward and "sit back" for the squat, keeping your head up and bending your knees. Lean your weight forward and place your hands on the floor, inside, outside or in front of your feet—whichever is more comfortable and gives you a nice, stable base.

3 Kick your feet straight back so that you're now in a push-up starting position, forming a nice line from your head to your feet. Keep your core tight to maintain an erect spine.

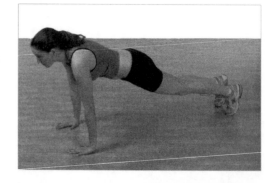

4 Inhale as you lower your torso toward the floor for a push-up. Stop when your body is 1–2 inches from the floor.

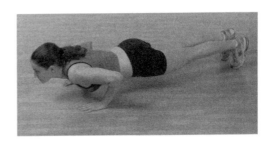

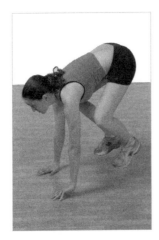

5 Exhaling, straighten your arms and propel your entire upper body off the floor while simultaneously bending your knees and bringing them toward your chest in order to plant your feet underneath you. You should end up back in the bottom position of a squat. Take a quick breath.

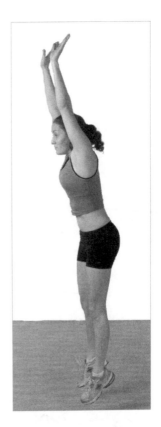

6 Swing your arms straight overhead, exhale and push off from your feet to jump straight up in the air as high as possible. Land with your knees slightly bent to absorb the impact. That's 1 rep.

Inchworm

This is a great full-body exercise and a perfect test for hamstring and lower back flexibility. In this motion-based exercise, you'll advance forward approximately 4 feet per repetition, so plan your exercise positioning accordingly.

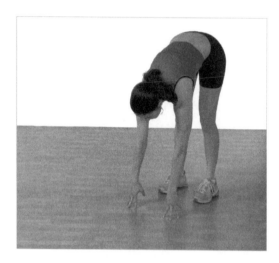

1 Stand with your feet about hip-width apart and fold over so that your hands touch the floor.

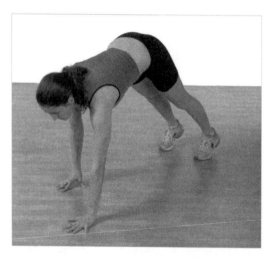

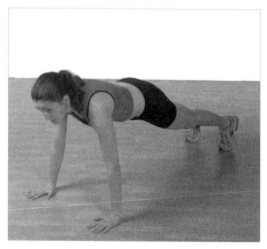

2–3 Keeping your hands firmly on the floor to balance your weight, walk your hands out in front of you one at a time until you're at the top of a push-up. Hold for 3 seconds.

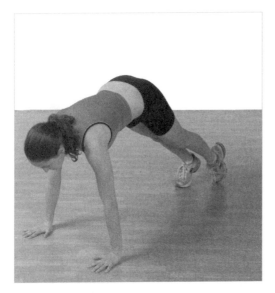
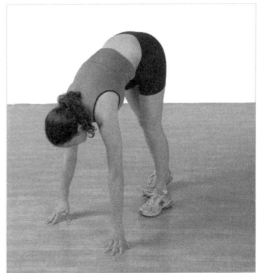

4—5 Keeping your hands firmly on the floor to balance your weight, "walk" your feet toward your head by taking very small steps on your toes. Imagine that your lower legs are bound together and you can only bend your feet at each ankle. As you continue walking your feet toward your head, your butt will rise and your body will form an inverse "V." When you've stretched your hamstrings, glutes and calves as far as you can, hold that position for 3 seconds. That's 1 rep.

RIPPED VARIATION: Every time you return to starting position, perform a proper-form push-up.

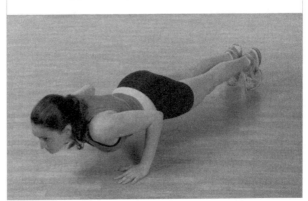

Wood Chop

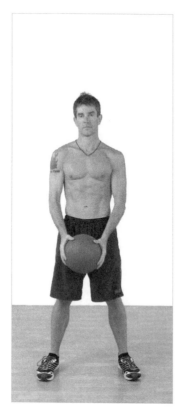 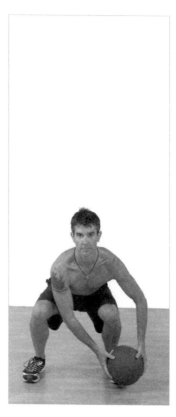 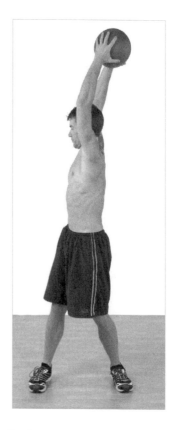

1 Stand tall with your feet shoulder-width apart, holding a medicine ball in front of you.

2 Lower your body into a squat until your knees are bent 90°, and bring the ball down to touch your left foot.

3 Stand tall, twisting your torso to the right and lifting your arms straight up over your head. Your left shoulder should be in front and you should be looking to the right.

Repeat to the other side.

MODIFICATION: This can also be done without a medicine ball.

J-Up

Named after its developer, Jason Warner, the J-up is one of the most amazing workouts you can get in 15 minutes. It consists of the following moves: squat, mountain climbers, push-up, air squat, pull-up and hanging leg raise—all in one! A pull-up bar is required. Position yourself directly under the bar with plenty of room around and above the pull-up apparatus. It's very important to orient yourself properly with the bar before starting so you can grip the bar when performing the pull-up and make sure that you don't hit your head on the bar when jumping up from the air squat. This is a very complicated exercise, so take your time to familiarize yourself with each and every part of the movement before attempting it at full speed.

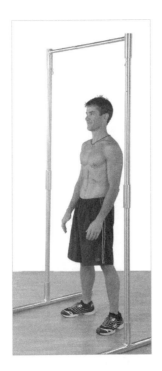 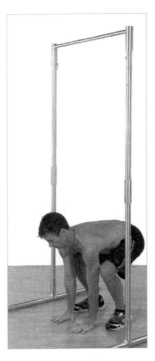 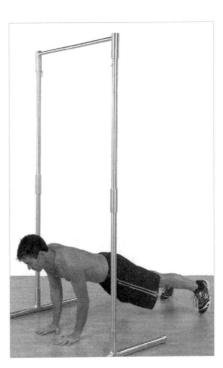

1 Stand beneath a pull-up bar with your feet slightly wider than your shoulders.

2–3 Lower your body into a squat. At the bottom of the squat, place both hands on the ground just in front of your feet and extend both feet straight back until your body is in push-up position, with your core engaged and body in a straight line from head to toe.

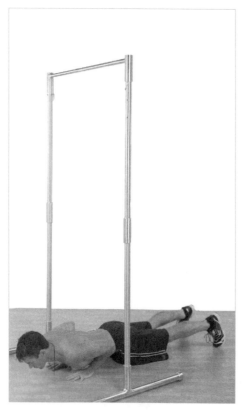 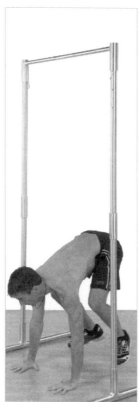 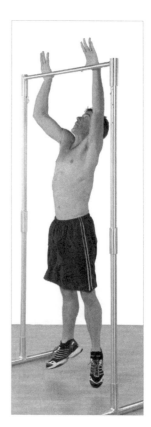

4 Lower your chest toward the floor.

5 When your chest is about 3 inches from the floor, use your arms, shoulders and chest to explosively push up your torso so that your hands leave the ground; simultaneously pull your feet back under your body into the bottom squat position with your knees bent.

6 Raise your hands directly overhead and perform an air squat, jumping straight up to grab the pull-up bar with your preferred grip (see Pull-Up Grip Variations, page 71).

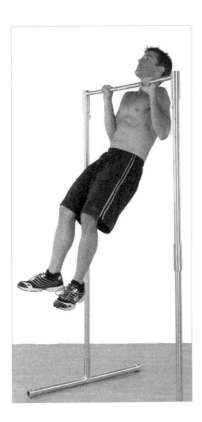 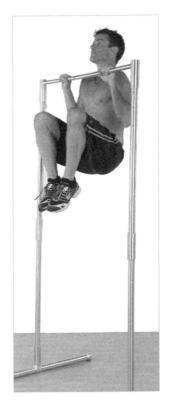 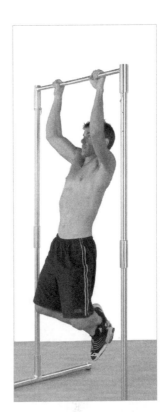

7 Use your upward momentum to pull your chest up to the bar.

8 Pull your elbows in to your body and hold that position while you raise both knees toward your chest. Don't swing when raising your legs; you'll activate your core a lot to keep your body straight, pull your knees up as straight as possible and "touch" the bar. Due to the differences in torso size and flexibility, some of you won't be able to touch your knees to the bar; just bring your knees up as far as you can and be careful not to hit your elbows!

9 Extend both legs beneath you, release the bar and drop your feet to the floor with your knees bent to absorb the impact. That's 1 rep.

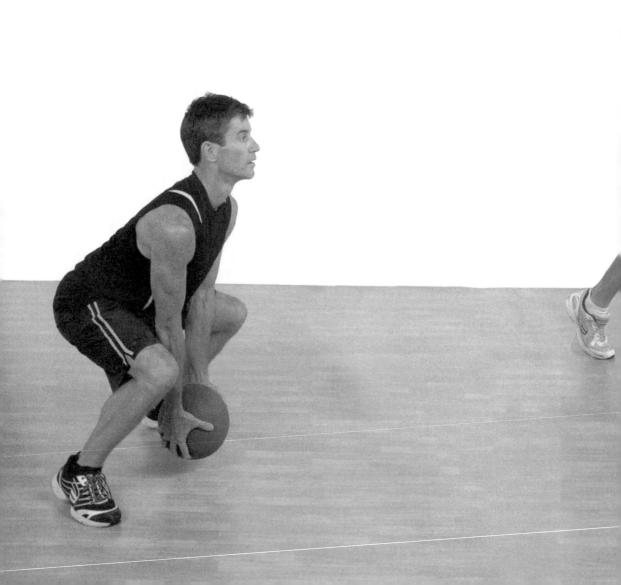

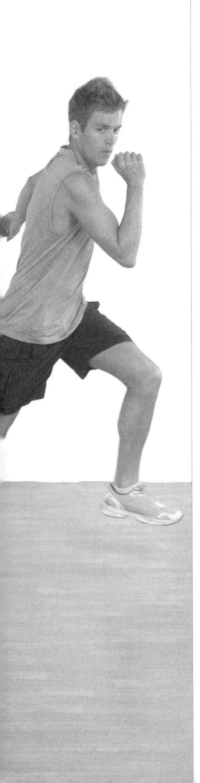

IAPPENDIX

Beyond the Program

So what do you do after you've achieved your lean, ripped body? The beauty of the *7 Weeks to Getting Ripped* program is that you now know all the exercises you need to strengthen and shred your body and can do them at any time! With all the moves you've learned combined with the cardio components and games, there are literally millions of exercise combinations you can use to build your own routines. Get creative and mix things up from week to week. You'll be amazed by how much fun you can have while getting fit. Want to challenge yourself to new goals in the routine? Add an additional set to each workout or double the cardio components—there are no bad combinations as long as you take at least one day off between workouts and don't overtrain.

Full-Body Exercises: A Complete Workout All by Themselves

Multijoint movements, commonly called compound exercises, are an efficient way to get a full-body workout done in less time. In this book we've covered many exercises that use your bodyweight and natural movements to achieve a complete workout. These exercises (squats, pull-ups, wood chops, in & outs, etc.) can be combined or modified to build strength and muscle quickly. To put it in a phrase, "The more joints that are worked, the more muscle fibers are activated and the better your results will be."

Okay, I understand the whole "multiple muscle" thing, but how does this make me stronger and leaner?

There are many factors that make compound exercises extremely effective at building a lean, ripped body. Here's a quick overview:

- By activating more muscle fibers, you place a greater demand on your body and rapidly consume more energy than when performing isolation movements. This in turn has a metabolic effect, helping you burn fat more quickly.

- When you activate multiple muscle groups by moving on one or more planes, you also stimulate and strengthen a great deal of stabilizing muscles.

- Real-life activities don't happen while sitting on a bench lifting a weight on a cable—natural movements are on multiple planes using multiple muscles at the same time. Training with compound movements improves performance in athletics as well as regular daily activity.

- Multijoint movements are extremely efficient, activating more muscle fibers in less time than when performing multiple isolation exercises.

Here are a few of my favorite multijoint "advanced" movements that aren't noted in the programs in this book but can be found in the exercises section (Part III). Give them a try!

AROUND-THE-WORLD MULE KICK MOUNTAIN CLIMBERS
(PAGE 101) As a marathoner, my hips always seem to be one of the first things to hurt during long mileage, and I needed to find an exercise I liked that would work my hips on multiple planes. I'm not a huge fan of sitting on a hip abductor machine, and the singular plane doesn't replicate the running motion too well, in my opinion. So I developed "Around-the-World Mule Kick Mountain Climbers" (in retrospect, I could've come up with a more clever name as an advanced variation of the mountain climber). This exercise combines a series of moves (plank, mountain climbers, mule kicks) and adds a hip movement on three different planes. My glutes, hips and core really get a workout from doing this exercise, I hope you like it, too! When I'm

doing the program, I'll swap a dozen or so of these in place of standard mountain climbers.

INCHWORM (PAGE 104) This is a complex strength-building locomotion exercise (like walking lunges, bear crawl, spiderman and others) in which you move forward to finish in a different location. When I'm doing the 7 Weeks to Getting Ripped program, occasionally I'll replace a set of push-ups with 10 of the advanced version of the inchworms. This is one of those exercises that never fails to get a couple of curious looks when I'm in the gym and "doing the worm."

J-UP (PAGE 107) Named after its creator Jason Warner, the J-up is an all-in-one, full-body, total-workout exercise. It's been described by some as the "perfect exercise," and once you master it you'll agree! The J-up is an extreme compound exercise that combines all of the "Power 4" moves (pull-up, squat, push-up, plank) and then increases the difficulty by making two of the moves plyometric. Essentially, the J-up is a complete full-body circuit workout rolled into one exercise.

While on the surface it may sound simple to combine all these exercises, there are certain nuances to the form of each move that you need to master separately before combining them into one series of movements. Foot position on your squats is extremely important, as is bent knees on landing back on the ground after

> Interested in more exercises that didn't make it in print? Check out 7weekstogettingripped.com, where we'll continue to add exercises, tips, tricks and techniques.

the pull-up and knee raise. This intense series will require some practice to master hand and foot position and control your body in all the different phases, from floor to bar and back again.

We've perfected this move over the course of a couple years at different gyms and parks by using pull-up bars, the top bar of a Smith machine, jungle gyms, etc. Practice it on a secure bar at home and then rock it out with high intensity at a gym. You'll be absolutely amazed at how many people ask you what the move is and how to do it. When Jason and I did 100 each, a small group of people watched and cheered us on at our local gym.

Maintaining Your Ripped Physique

One of my favorite maintenance workouts involves devoting one day a week (most often Wednesday) to high-intensity training intervals (HIIT). I'll run up a hill for 30 seconds and then jog/walk back down about for 1 minute and repeat for 20 minutes. After 5 minutes of resting, stretching and re-hydrating, I run for 30 minutes at a moderate pace, trying to keep my heart rate at around 125 bpm (see "Finding Your Target Heart Rate" on page 127).

The other two days of the week (usually Monday or Friday), I'll pick a routine from the book, jog to a local park and complete three to four rounds before jogging back. On Saturday or Sunday I'll either play a few of the games with friends, challenge myself with a couple rounds of "Hot Corner" or play some organized sports.

Keep your routine flexible and mix it up as often as you can. Select one day a month and challenge yourself with as many J-ups as you can do or retake the "Power 4" test. You have all the tools to stay fit and healthy—it's really up to you how you use them. Numerous studies show that people who stay active live a longer, happier life. Use what you've learned in this book to keep yourself motivated to stay fit and inspire others to do the same. It's extremely easy to become a "fitness role model" to others once you have success; make sure you take that role seriously and help others to achieve their fitness goals.

EATING TO GET—AND STAY—RIPPED

As we covered earlier, to get ripped you should eat approximately 1 gram of lean protein per pound of your desired weight. If your goal is to be 165 lb at the end of this program, then you want to eat 165 grams of protein a day. Good sources of protein include lean beef and poultry, eggs, fish, yogurt (especially Greek), tempeh, nuts and legumes, quinoa, oats and milk. Eating chicken and fish is generally considered the quickest and healthiest way to increase your protein intake: 4 ounces of grilled chicken contains about 32 grams of protein. To get enough protein, you may need to supplement with some protein powder. Any whey protein will do—egg or milk—but be careful of the amount of sugar the powder contains. Optimally, you should try to find a protein powder that has less than 1 gram of sugar for every gram of protein (e.g., 24 grams of protein will have less than 2.4 grams of sugar).

So, if up to 50% of our daily intake is protein, does that mean carbs and fats can split the remaining 50%? Simply put, yes, provided you obtain good sources of each.

Good fats—mostly unsaturated—include avocados; oils like olive, safflower, corn, peanut and coconut; poultry; seeds; nuts; fish and flaxseed; eggs; and lean red meat. Avoid processed trans fats altogether, like those found in snack foods, margarine, prepared desserts and fast food. Try to keep fats to 20–25% of your daily nutrient intake.

Carbohydrates are an important source of energy, but you need to separate the good carbs from the bad. The best carbohydrates come from green leafy vegetables, either raw or steamed. The more you cook veggies, the more minerals and vitamins are lost. All other vegetables, beans, legumes, nuts and seeds are also healthy carb sources. Whole-grain breads and pastas are okay in moderation, but quite often contain extra sugars and other less-healthy grains. Because breads and pastas are manufactured foods it's important that you check the nutritional facts on the label before you buy.

Warm-Ups & Stretches

As we discussed on page 30, since you'll be pushing, pressing and lifting your bodyweight, it's very important to warm up before you stretch. Stretching prior to warming up can cause more damage than good to muscles, ligaments and joints. When your muscles are cold, they're far less pliable and you don't receive any benefit from stretching prior to warming up. Below are some dynamic warm-ups that'll get your heart rate up, loosen tight muscles and prepare you for your workout.

After your workout, stretching will help you reduce soreness, increase range of motion and flexibility within a joint or muscle, and prepare your body for any future workouts. Stretching immediately postexercise while your muscles are still warm allows your muscles to return to their full range of motion (which gives you more flexibility gains) and reduces the chance of injury or fatigue in the hours or days after an intense workout.

It's important to remember that even when you're warm and loose, you should never "bounce" during stretching. Keep your movements slow and controlled. The stretches in this section should be performed in order to optimize your recovery. Remember to exhale as you perform every deep stretch and rest 30 seconds in between each stretch.

Warm-Ups

Arm Circle

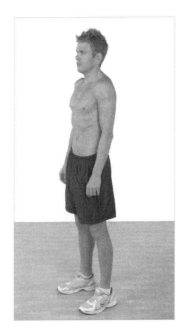 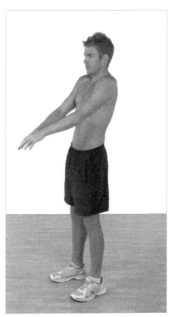 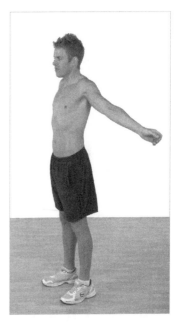

1 Stand with your feet shoulder-width apart.

2–3 Move both arms in a complete circle forward 5 times and then backward 5 times.

Lumber Jack

1 Stand with your feet shoulder-width apart and extend your hands overhead with elbows locked, fingers interlocked, and palms up.

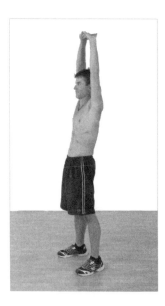

2 Bend forward at the waist and try to put your hands on the ground (like you're chopping wood).

Raise up and repeat.

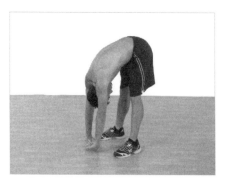

Side Bend

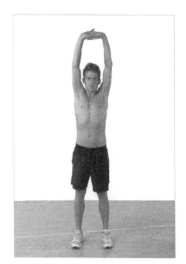

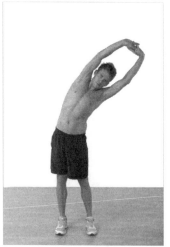

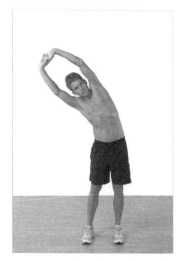

1 Stand with your feet shoulder-width apart and extend your hands overhead

with elbows locked, fingers interlocked and palms up.

2-3 Bend side to side.

Around the World

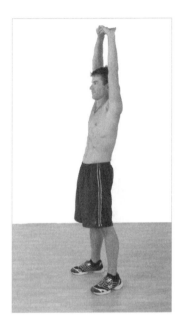

1 Stand with your feet shoulder-width apart and extend your hands overhead with elbows locked, fingers interlocked, and palms up. Keep your arms straight the entire time.

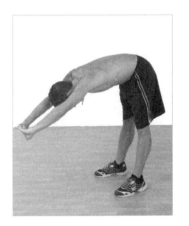 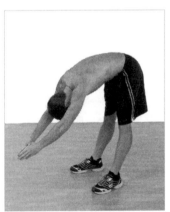 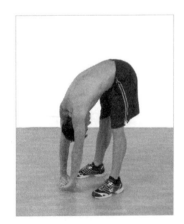

2–4 Bending at the hips, bring your hands down toward your right leg, and in a continuous circular motion bring your hands toward your toes, then toward your left leg and then return your hands overhead and bend backward.

Repeat three times, then change directions.

Barn Doors

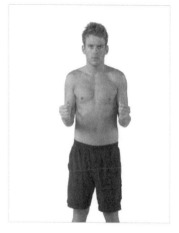

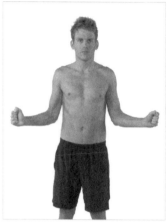

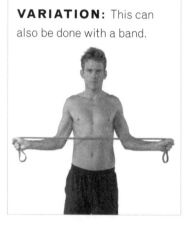

VARIATION: This can also be done with a band.

1 Stand with your feet shoulder-width apart with your arms tight against your sides. Bend your arms 90° so that your forearms extend forward and are parallel to the floor. Grip your hands like you have a rubber band between them.

2 Keeping your forearms parallel to the floor, squeeze your shoulder blades together and pull your hands apart to the sides.

Do 10–12 repetitions.

Chest Fly

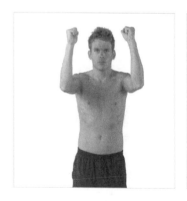

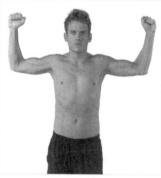

1 Assume the Barn Doors position (above) with your hands in front of your torso, then raise your hands and elbows straight up, maintaining the 90° angle until your elbows are at shoulder height.

2 Squeezing your shoulder blades together, pull your hands away from each other until your hands are parallel to your ears.

Do 10–12 repetitions.

Marching Twist

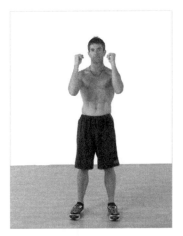 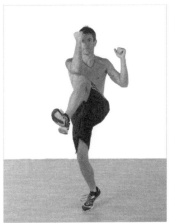 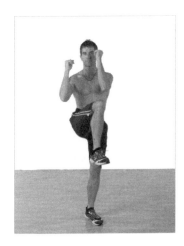

1 Stand tall with your feet shoulder-width apart. Bring your arms in front of you and bend your elbows 90°.

2 Twist your torso to the right and raise your left knee to your right elbow.

3 Repeat with your right knee and left elbow. A little hop with the bottom foot helps you keep your momentum going from leg to leg.

Do 10 reps on each leg.

Jumping Jacks

1 Stand tall with your feet together and arms extended along your sides, palms facing forward.

2 Jump 6–12 inches off the ground and simultaneously spread your feet apart an additional 20–30 inches while extending your hands directly overhead.

Jump 6–12 inches off the ground and return your hands and feet to the starting position. Do 10 reps.

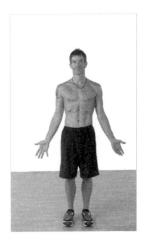 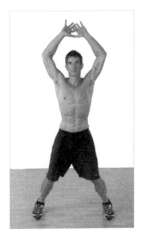

Stretches

Forearm & Wrist

Begin the stretch gently and allow your forearms to relax before stretching them to their full range of motion.

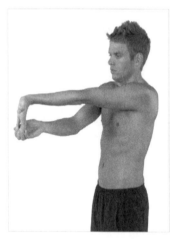 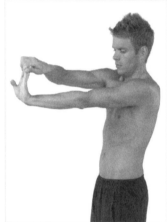

1 Stand with your feet shoulder-width apart and extend both arms straight out in front of you. Keep your back straight. Turn your right wrist to the sky and grasp your right fingers from below with your left hand. Slowly pull your fingers back toward your torso with your left hand; hold for 10 seconds.

2 Swap arms and repeat.

Shoulders

1 Stand with your feet shoulder-width apart and bring your left arm across your chest. Support your left elbow with the crook of your right arm by raising your right arm to 90°. Gently pull your left arm to your chest while maintaining proper posture (straight back, wide shoulders). Don't round or hunch your shoulders. Hold your arm to your chest for 10 seconds.

2 Release and switch arms.

After you've done both sides, shake your hands out for 5–10 seconds.

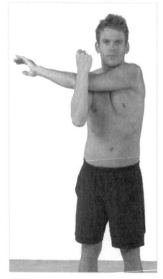 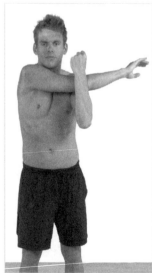

Shoulders & Upper Back

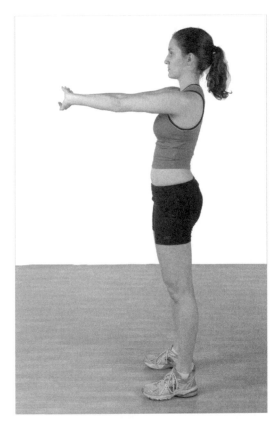 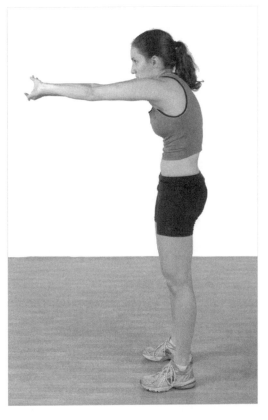

1 Stand with your feet shoulder-width apart and extend both arms straight out in front of you. Interlace your fingers and turn your palms to face away from your body. Keep your back straight.

2 Reach your palms away from your body. Exhale as you push your palms straight out from your body by pushing through your shoulders and upper back. Allow your neck to bend naturally as you round your upper back. Continue to reach your hands and stretch for 10 seconds.

Rest for 30 seconds then repeat. After you've done the second set, shake your arms out for 10 seconds to your sides to return blood to the fingers and forearm muscles.

Chest

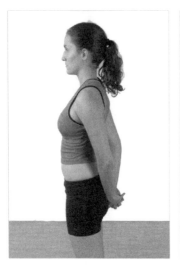 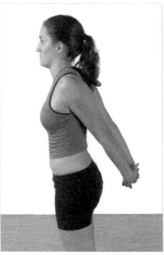

1 Clasp your hands together behind your lower back with palms facing each other.

2 Keeping an erect posture and your arms as straight as possible, gently pull your arms away from your back, straight out behind you. Keep your shoulders down. Hold for 10 seconds.

Rest for 30 seconds and repeat.

Arms

1 Stand with your feet shoulder-width apart. Maintaining a straight back, grab your elbows with the opposite hand. Slowly raise your arms until they're slightly behind your head. Keeping your right hand on your left elbow, drop your left hand to the top of your right shoulder blade. Gently push your left elbow down with your right hand, and hold for 10 seconds.

Rest for 10 seconds and then repeat with opposite arms.

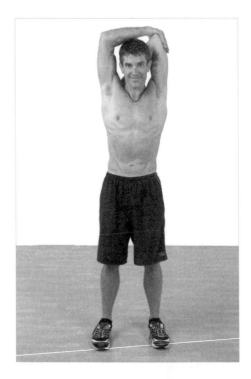

Lower Back

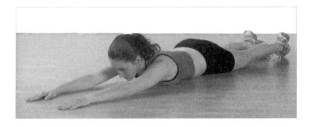

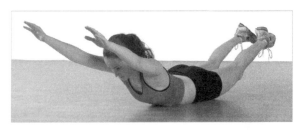

1 Lying face-down on your stomach, extend your arms along the floor above your head, palms on the ground. Keeping your knees straight, extend your legs behind you, keeping your feet close together and your toes on the ground.

2 In a slow, controlled motion, contract your lower back (erector spinae) and raise your arms and legs 6–8 inches off the floor. Hold for 5 seconds.

Lower slowly back to starting position. Repeat slowly 10 times.

Neck

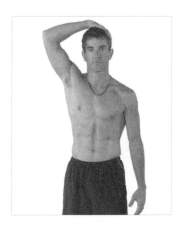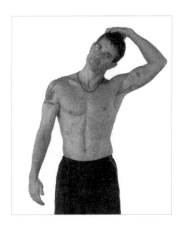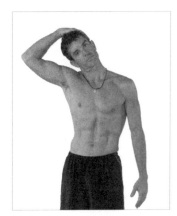

1 Standing like a soldier (with your back straight, shoulders square and chest raised), slowly lower your left ear to your left shoulder. To increase the stretch, you may use your left hand to gently pull your head toward your shoulder. Hold for 5–10 seconds.

2–3 Slowly roll your chin to your chest and then lower your right ear to your right shoulder. Again, you may use your hand to enhance the stretch. Hold for 5–10 seconds.

Return your head to normal position and then tilt back slightly and look straight up. Hold for 5–10 seconds.

Cardio & Games

"Ugh. Cardio." To most fitness enthusiasts, cardio work is just a boring, tedious time-eater at the end of a workout. Getting the most out of your cardio, however, doesn't mean you need to spend an hour on an oversized hamster wheel just to fulfill a quota. Anything that involves you getting active and raising your heart rate counts.

Use the following list of cardio components as a guide for raising your heart rate, building your endurance, strength and flexibility, and burning more calories and fat. Be inventive: Toss a medicine ball against a wall or with a partner, jump rope, hop over cones, bound up some stairs or, my personal favorite, dance with your kids. Like the saying goes, "Dance like no one is watching."

At the end of each daily workout is a basic idea of how much time you should put in for cardio. It's not set in stone and varies greatly on the exercise you choose and your intensity. The more effort you put into your cardio, the more quickly you'll be done. Mix and match a few different moves, like jumping rope and shadow boxing, to work your whole body, and you'll be sufficiently smoked and ready for the shower before you know it.

Team or individual sports also count as excellent cardio. Sometimes the best way to get a great workout, as well as renew the spirit, is to grab a partner and engage in some friendly competition. Play some one-on-one basketball or shoot around by yourself to get a good burn. For more ideas, check out "Fitness Games" on page 130. The key to games, both winning and getting a great workout, is intensity— the harder you compete, the better the results and the more fun you'll have, fueling the desire to do it again.

All of the games provide a bit of everything you'll need to get ripped so don't fret over which is best; just find those that work for you and have fun with them. As time goes on, create your own and have even more fun!

Safety note: If you're outdoors, especially near traffic, always be aware of your surroundings!

FINDING YOUR TARGET HEART RATE

In order to optimize fat burning, it's important for you to calculate your resting heart rate (RHR) and use that to find your target heart rate (THR).

To calculate your maximum heart rate (MHR) (the theoretical maximum beats per minute your heart can physically handle):

$$220 - YOUR\ AGE = MHR$$

To calculate 60% of your MHR to keep your cardio in the fat-burning zone (or THR):

$$220 - YOUR\ AGE \times DESIRED\ \% = THR$$

In order to make your THR percentage even more accurate, you need to know your resting heart rate (RHR). Take your HR first thing in the morning when you wake up and use this formula:

$$(220 - YOUR\ AGE - RHR) \times DESIRED\ \% + RHR = THR$$

Note that you subtract your RHR before multiplying by the desired HR% and then add your RHR back in.

Cardio Components

JUMPING JACKS

You gym teacher was right—you'll use this exercise for the rest of your life. Don't settle for just a boring old set of jumping jacks—add a twist, lunge or side-step and make it a full-body move. Check out Marching Twists below for another way to mix it up.

SHADOW BOXING

The good news about shadow boxing is that your shadow won't be punching you back, although after about three minutes of vigorous punches and footwork you might be wishing for someone to knock

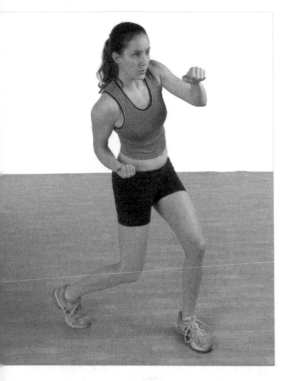

you out! Try timing yourself for a minute at normal intensity and then punch like crazy for the next 30 seconds. It's amazing how exhausting yet cathartic it can be to get your aggressions out.

JUMPING ROPE

We all know that boxers jump rope as a way to improve their agility, timing and cardiovascular system, as well as keep them lean, so why don't you try it, too? There are many different variations like speed-step, crisscross, side swing, double under…so get a rope and get jumping!

STAIRS

Most buildings have these contraptions and most folks walk right past to grab the elevator. Since no one else seems to use them, make these your playground. Sprint up, walk down; take two steps at a time; bunny hop up with both feet together… whatever works for you as long as you're careful and don't take a tumble.

MARCHING TWISTS   *page 99*

Can you do the can-can? With your arms at 90°, twist your torso and raise your left knee to your right elbow. Repeat with your right knee and left elbow… and put a little rhythm into it! A little hop with the bottom foot helps you keep your momentum going from leg to leg. Start slow and work up the intensity, even throw in some intervals (See Music Intervals on the next page) to really raise your heart rate. Feel free to get creative, work in some lunges, jumping jacks and other moves and create your own aerobics routine!

MEDICINE BALL TOSSES

The medicine ball, long a tool for doing core exercises, is fabulous as a game prop whether you do tosses by yourself by throwing the ball against the ground/wall or toss it back and forth with a partner. I recommend starting with a lighter weight and progressing to a heavier one as you're able. (See page 130 for examples.)

AIR SQUATS   *page 94*

These are exactly as the name implies— squats where you catch some air.

BURPEES   *page 102*

This great, full-body workout can be done anywhere to work up a sweat and target your arms, chest, glutes, quads, hamstrings, calves and core. To spice it up, add a push-up, plank or mountain climbers when you're in push-up position. If you're ready to really get nuts, the J-Up (page 107) is the big brother (we're talking Andre the Giant big) of burpees.

SPRINT INTERVALS

Choose a few different spots no farther than 25 yards apart. Set down a marker and alternate jogging, bounding, high knees, butt-kickers, crossover side bounds and sprinting between each point. If you're on a sports field or a flat, grass-covered surface, try sprinting barefoot, which has helped me strengthen my feet, ankles and calves. Take it easy at first! (See "Hot Corner" on page 134 for more details.)

TREADMILL INCLINE INTERVALS

Hop on a treadmill and start at 0 incline and a moderate speed. Every 2 minutes, raise the incline .5 and raise the speed by .5. See how high you can go! Also try doing Music Intervals (below) by raising the speed/incline each time your songs hit the chorus—be creative. *Safety note:* Never exceed a speed that you can handle and make sure you're comfortable before attempting any high inclines and rates of speed.

HIT THE DECK

Run in place for 30 seconds, drop to the ground with your chest flat on the floor, perform an explosive push-up and return to your feet and repeat. Decrease duration 5 seconds each repetition until you hit 0.

MUSIC INTERVALS

This can be done on any cardio equipment and also works great with all calisthenics and sprints. Pop your earphones in and crank the tunes. During the verses of the song, perform your exercise at moderate pace; when the chorus comes in, up your intensity to 80%. If you're lucky enough to have a guitar solo, try and hit 100%!

Fitness Games

Here are just a few ideas to get you started. Visit our website 7weekstogetting ripped.com for additional tosses that didn't make it into print.

MEDICINE BALL LONGEST TOSS

The goal is to create as much distance between you and your partner by tossing a medicine ball back and forth using a variety of throwing techniques. This involves a lot of jumping, squatting and twisting, so make sure you're warmed up before attempting any of them. *Safety note:* NEVER try to catch a thrown medicine ball. Let it bounce, as all the instructions say to do!

Number of players: 2

Description: Using 4 cones, place 2 cones side by side and the other 2 about 10 feet apart. Stand next to a pair of cones and face your partner, who's standing next to the other pair of cones. Choose who goes first. Begin tossing the ball as far as you can toward your partner's cones.

Your partner will move one of his cones to that spot; he makes his next throw from there, whether it's farther or closer than the original 10 feet. Keep the other cone at the original 10-foot starting position. Each of you will perform the 10 tosses below to determine a winner for each round. The winner is the person whose cone is still closest to the other cone in its original starting position.

A match is played by alternating through the following tosses:

TOSS 1: *Overhead Forward* With your arms extended straight overhead with the ball between both hands, keep both feet planted (no steps allowed) and pointed directly at your partner's cone. Lean back slightly, engaging your core and lower back muscles. Do not bend your elbows to bring the ball behind the top of your head; your arms should always remain straight. Rapidly contract your core, bring your whole upper body forward and release the ball. You should be throwing the ball with your core, not your arms.

TOSS 1

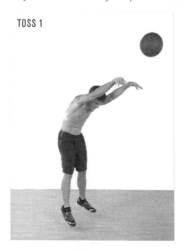

TOSS 2

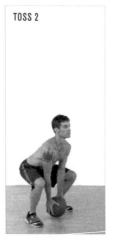

TOSS 3

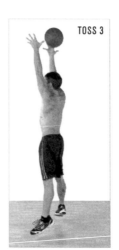

TOSSES 4 & 5

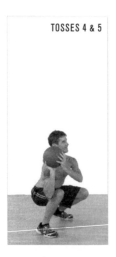

TOSS 2: *Underhand Forward* With your feet pointing directly at your partner, assume a squat position with the ball on the ground between your feet. Put your hands under the ball and shovel the ball forward as you explode upward. Your arms are just guiding the ball; you should be throwing the ball with the explosive force of your legs.

TOSS 3: *Underhand Backward* Start in a squat with your back facing your partner and explode upward, swinging the ball up over your head and throwing it behind you. This is traditionally responsible for the longest throws and engages your entire body. Feel free to let out a strong grunt when you explode from the ground.

TOSSES 6 & 7

If you're competing for distance, limit the height of the arc.

TOSSES 4 & 5: *Shot Put* Place the ball in one hand next to your shoulder with your palm up and use your other hand to steady it. Your feet should point directly at your partner and in the direction you'll be tossing. Squat straight down (don't twist) and, when you've reached the deepest part of your squat, explode upward, leave your feet and toss the ball as far as you can toward your partner's cone. While this move uses a lot of arm muscle, you'll be using far more force from your legs to launch the ball. Alternate between hands for throws.

TOSSES 6 & 7: *Shot-Put Twist* Start with your feet pointed 90° in relation to your partner and the direction you intend to throw the ball. Hold the ball in your hand with your palm up and steady it with your other hand while you lower into a squat and twist to the side holding the ball. At the bottom of the squat, you should have twisted far enough so that the ball is almost completely behind your shoulder. Uncoil while you're exploding upward and throw the ball completely across your body toward your partner's cone. This throw uses a lot of leg and arm strength, but also the torsion of your core, to chuck the ball. Alternate between hands for throws.

TOSS 8: *Bounce Pass* With your arms extended straight overhead with the ball between both hands, keep both feet planted (no steps allowed) and lean back slightly, engaging your core and lower back muscles. Do not bend your elbows to bring the ball behind the top of your head; your arms should always remain straight. Rapidly contract your core, bring your whole upper body forward and release the ball, throwing it as hard as you can into the ground to get it to bounce. You should be throwing the ball with your core, not your arms. The distance is measured by where the ball stops rolling. One rule: The ball must hit the ground within 5 feet of where you're standing.

TOSSES 9 & 10: *One-Legged Shot Put*

With ball in hand, stand with both feet pointed at your target and lift the foot opposite from the ball off the ground. Squat down as far as you can without letting your "up" foot touch and launch upward from your one leg, extending your arm to release the ball. This is an excellent move to improve your balance and strength, but also a great way to end the round as one of you is bound to lose your balance and not toss the ball very far. If your raised foot touches the ground, it's a foul and you must re-shoot. Alternate between hands for each toss.

TOSS & RUN

Number of players: 1

Description: Throw a medicine ball as far as possible using an underhand technique. Once the ball is released, sprint after it as fast as you can. Gather the medicine ball and throw again until you've reached the end of the field. Repeat with no rest, going back down the field to the starting position. Repeat as desired. Alternate medicine ball throws, too.

LEAPFROG

There's no winner or loser in this game—just exhaust yourself and your partner.

Number of players: 2

Description: Both players start at an end line or cone. One person starts the game by throwing the medicine ball as far as possible using an overhand forward toss. Both players sprint after the ball as soon as it's released. The nontossing player gathers the ball and throws it farther down the field. The original tosser will already be sprinting past him to catch up with the

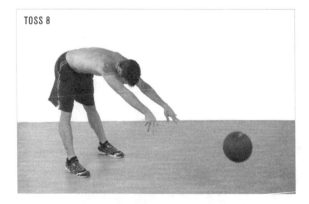

TOSS 8

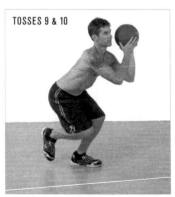

TOSSES 9 & 10

newly thrown ball. Repeat up and down the field, changing directions as needed.

Alternate each toss as follows: overhand forward, underhand forward, shot put.

OUT & BACK SPRINTS

Win the game by being the last one standing.

Number of players: 2+

Description: Start with 2 players side by side at a pair of cones. One player tosses the ball using either an overhand forward, underhand forward or shot put toss. The other player sprints after the ball, picks it up over his head and sprints back with the ball overhead. Be careful and keep a good grip on the ball over your head. When the sprinter makes it back to the starting position, switch roles (if you have more than 2 players, just rotate so everyone gets a turn). The first one to call it quits loses.

BALL SPRINTS

Footballs, soccer balls, tennis balls, rugby balls or even Australian rules footballs—we've experimented with each and love them all. The games you find here are a smattering of what's possible when you use your imagination with what you have on hand. The rule to remember in this section is throw or kick the ball really far and run like hell after it.

PUNTERS

This is one of our "go-to" games to make sprinting and speedwork fun while still having an element of game play. An absolute blast with anywhere from 2 to 4 people (any more seems to get too chaotic), this is best played on a soccer field, but improvisation will allow nearly any grassy field to suffice.

Number of players: 2–4

Description: Everyone starts at the end line near a soccer goal. One person punts a football as far as he can, the rest sprint after the ball. The first person to touch the ball gains possession and the right to attempt to score a goal. From where the ball was touched, the player gaining possession has two tries to score a goal by punting the ball downfield and then into the goal. Three points will be awarded if a goal is scored in one kick, one point if in two kicks. After a goal attempt is completed, a new round starts with the person gaining possession in the previous round as the new punter. An American football bounces so erratically you never know what'll end up in the net! To make the game a little more predictable, use a soccer ball. To make it more international, use a rugby ball.

TENNIS BALL TOSSES

I use this whenever I need to get a workout but am not motivated to do sprints.

Number of players: 1

Description: In any open, grassy field, throw a tennis ball as high and far as you can. As soon as you release it, sprint after it and try to catch it before it hits the ground. If you catch it before it bounces once, that's 3 points. If it bounces once, give yourself 1 point. If it bounces more than once, you get zero for that toss. Play against yourself to 21 for a killer workout.

HOT CORNER

Ready for a great workout that's essentially circuit training with a race element? Find a soccer field and a buddy and get ready!

Number of players: 1–8

Description: This is ideally played on a soccer field, though anywhere you can mark off stations will suffice. Break down the field into sections, each one for a specific movement. See the diagram opposite for a sample breakdown. This game/race is all about intensity, so get creative! Add a flight of stairs, a hill or anything else that strikes your fancy.

Station 1 is the starting and ending point. At each point on the field designated in the diagram, perform a specific move-

ment type as quickly as possible and then move on to the next segment.

Stations 1–5 : Push-up movements

Station 1: 10 Standard push-ups
Station 2: 10 Diamond push-ups
Station 3: 10 Wide push-ups
Station 4: 10 Narrow push-ups
Station 5: 10 Standard push-ups

Run 1–5 : Running movements

Run 1: Run backward from Station 1 to Core 1
Run 2: High knees/plyo skips from Core 1 to Station 2
Run 3: Side to side from Station 2 to Station 3. At the halfway mark of Run 3, rotate 180 degrees to use both sides of your body.
Run 4: Butt kicks from Station 3 to Core 2
Run 5: Lunges from Core 2 to Station 4
SPRINT!: Explode up from the last push-up and go!

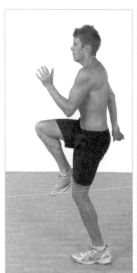
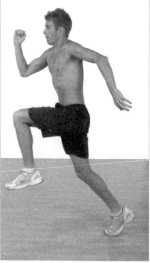
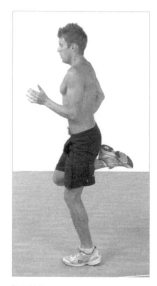

High knees are also known as plyometric skips.

Butt kicks

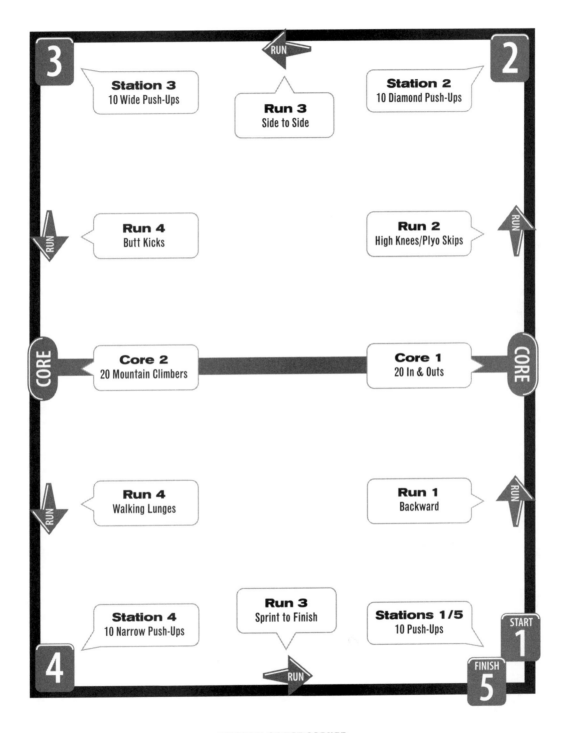

DIAGRAM OF HOT CORNER

Core 1 & 2 : Core movements

Core 1: 20 In & out crunches

Core 2: 20 Mountain climbers

Everyone starts at Station 1, which would be a corner of the soccer field—it's both the starting and ending line. As soon as "GO" is yelled, everyone drops and does 10 standard push-ups. When you finish the push-ups, run backward to the center of the soccer field for Core 1 (20 in & out crunches). When you finish the crunches, bound down the field to Station 2 doing high knees (also known as plyometric skips). Perform 10 diamond push-ups at Station 3 and then start side-to-sides down the end line of the soccer field (you'll be passing directly in front of the goal). Once you reach the halfway point (the middle of the goal), turn around 180 degrees and finish the rest of the way using your other side.

The second half of this game is where it gets real. Consider the first half a gentle warm-up!

At Station 3 perform 10 wide push-ups, then run down the field performing butt kicks as fast as you can toward Core 2. At Core 2, do 20 mountain climbers (10 each side). Once you're finished with mountain climbers, do forward walking lunges until you reach Station 4, where you'll do 10 narrow push-ups. On your last push-up, explode up into a full sprint across the soccer field to Station 5. As soon as you cross the boundary line at Station 5, drop and do 10 standard push-ups. The first person to complete all this is the winner.

To really shred up fast, that's just the first of a few rounds of the Hot Corner. After completing the first round, rest 3–5 minutes and hydrate before your next round. If you're using the right amount of intensity, I wouldn't recommend more than one round until you're already in great shape and your body can take it. Trust me when I say that the Hot Corner will be one of the most fun but also hardest 4 minutes of your life.

Remember: The Hot Corner is also a great individual workout! Get out and get motivated for a fantastic workout!

Prep-Level Program

Welcome to the Prep program, a fantastic place to start and an awesome opportunity for men and women of all fitness levels to build the full-body strength they'll need to complete the programs in Part II. The Prep level builds progressively over three weeks and packs a lot of training and learning into that short span of time. It's imperative that you use this program to not only build your strength and stamina, but also to master all of the movements so you can perform them repeatedly with good form. A great deal of people will repeat the Prep program until they're ready to make the leap into Level I.

You'll find instructions for the exercises either after the Prep program test on page 142 or in Part III. The Prep program is a kick-off for newcomers to full-body workouts work but it also works very well as a maintenance program for staying in shape after you've completed Level I or Level II. This program can double as an effective "on the road" workout that you can do virtually anywhere—a hotel room, on a camping trip, even backstage.

Prep Program Tips

Take this workout at your own pace if you're new to working out or coming back after some time away. **DO NOT OVERDO IT!** (Did I make that bold enough?) You WILL be sore for 1–2 days after your first few workouts, and if you overdo it you'll miss subsequent workouts. This happens to nearly everyone when they start a workout regimen—don't let it happen to you.

The goal with assisted pull-ups and knee/wall push-ups is to get you strong enough to perform the movements without assistance by the end of the Prep program. For some people it'll take longer to achieve the minimum (5) pull-ups for the Level I program. Don't get discouraged! You can repeat the Prep program as many times as you'd like to build your strength and increase the intensity on the other exercises. Here's a little secret: The Prep program will get you stronger and more ripped, too!

Huge gains in strength and fitness are nice but about as realistic as expecting the Tooth Fairy slipping a C-note under your pillow. As long as you put in the effort, you'll get results. Persistence and intensity along with the workout programs in this book are all you need to get ripped.

Nothing is more motivating than having a "before" picture, whether you post it on your fridge or keep it on your phone. It's really important to see where you were so after completing any program you can see your improvements.

You'll always miss some workouts, no matter how hard you try and prepare—life gets in the way. Don't be discouraged if you miss a day—just slide your routine back a day for the rest of the week and start again on Monday. If you missed a week, just restart the following Monday. Don't give up. The goal isn't "7 weeks"; it's all about you getting in the best shape of your life. Even if it takes six months of stops and starts, the end result is totally worth the effort!

Note: Rest and recovery are vital to the success of the programs and should be included as prescribed on the schedules. Remember also to warm up before your workout and stretch afterward! See pages 116–25 for ideas.

Prep Level

Week 1		Rest 2 minutes after every set (longer if required)			
Mon	*set 1*	4 Push-Ups	6 Squats	:30 Plank	3 Assisted Chin-Ups
	set 2	5 Push-Ups	5 Lunges per leg	3 Assisted Pull-Ups	8 In & Outs
	set 3	10 Wood Chops	16 Marching Twists	8 Mountain Climbers	—
	cardio	10 minutes cardio/game			
Tue		Rest			
Wed	*set 1*	3 Push-Ups	:20 Plank	10 Mountain Climbers	2 Assisted Pull-Ups
	set 2	6 Lunges w/ Twist per leg	10 Wood Chops	18 Marching Twists	8 Squats
	set 3	3 Assisted Chin-Ups	8 Hanging Leg Raises	8 Reverse Crunches	—
	cardio	10 minutes cardio/game			
Thu		Rest			
Fri	*set 1*	3 Assisted Pull-Ups	5 Push-Ups	8 Squats w/ Medicine Ball	12 Mountain Climbers
	set 2	10 Hanging Leg Raises	6 Lunges w/Twist per leg	5 Push-Ups	10 In & Outs
	set 3	3 Assisted Chin-Ups	12 Wood Chops	20 Marching Twists	8 Squats
	cardio	10 minutes cardio/game			
Sat		Rest			
Sun		Rest			

Note: Rest and recovery are vital to the success of the programs and should be included as prescribed on the schedules. Remember also to warm up before your workout and stretch afterward! See pages 116–25 for ideas.

Prep Level

Week 2		Rest 2 minutes after every set (longer if required)			
Mon	set 1	5 Assisted Chin-Ups	10 Squats	8 Push-Ups	:30 Plank
	set 2	14 Wood Chops	12 Mountain Climbers	20 Marching Twists	12 Jumping Jacks
	set 3	6 Push-Ups	:30 Plank	:15 Side Plank each side	10 Reverse Crunches
	cardio	10 minutes cardio/game			
Tue		Rest			
Wed	set 1	6 Assisted Pull-Ups	5 Push-Ups	8 Squats w/ Medicine Ball	10 Mountain Climbers
	set 2	10 Hanging Leg Raises	6 Lunges w/Twist per leg	5 Push-Ups	10 In & Outs
	set 3	2 Chin-Ups	12 Wood Chops	16 Marching Twists	8 Squats
	cardio	10 minutes cardio/game			
Thu		Rest			
Fri	set 1	8 Push-Ups	11 Squats	:30 Plank	6 Assisted Chin-Ups
	set 2	8 Push-Ups	8 Lunges w/Twist per leg	2 Pull-Ups	10 In & Outs
	set 3	14 Wood Chops	20 Marching Twists	12 Mountain Climbers	12 Jumping Jacks
	cardio	10 minutes cardio/game			
Sat		Rest			
Sun		Rest			

Note: Rest and recovery are vital to the success of the programs and should be included as prescribed on the schedules. Remember also to warm up before your workout and stretch afterward! See pages 116–25 for ideas.

Prep Level

Week 3		Rest 2 minutes after every set (longer if required)			
Mon	*set 1*	6 Assisted Pull-Ups	8 Push-Ups	12 Squats w/ Medicine Ball	14 Mountain Climbers
	set 2	12 Hanging Leg Raises	8 Lunges w/ Twist per leg	8 Push-Ups	10 Reverse Crunches
	set 3	3 Chin-Ups	14 Wood Chops	20 Marching Twists	:45 Plank
	cardio	10 minutes cardio/game			
Tue		Rest			
Wed	*set 1*	12 Hanging Leg Raises	8 Lunges w/Twist per leg	9 Push-Ups	12 In & Outs
	set 2	3 Pull-Ups	8 Push-Ups	14 Squats w/ Medicine Ball	16 Mountain Climbers
	set 3	3 Chin-Ups	16 Wood Chops	20 Marching Twists	12 Squats
	cardio	10 minutes cardio/game			
Thu		Rest			
Fri	*set 1*	4 Chin-Ups	14 Hanging Leg Raises	9 Lunges w/ Twist per leg	8 Push-Ups
	set 2	3 Pull-Ups	16 Squats	:45 Plank	8 Push-Ups
	set 3	3 Chin-Ups	14 Reverse Crunches	16 Mountain Climbers	18 Wood Chops
	cardio	10 minutes cardio/game			
Sat		Rest			
Sun		Rest			

Prep Program Test

Congratulations on completing the Prep program! Now is a great time to test your progress. Take at least 2 full days of rest and take the intro test of the "Power 4" moves again:

- **MAX NUMBER OF PULL-UPS**

  (2:00 rest, write down your results)

- **MAX NUMBER OF SQUATS**

  (2:00 rest, write down your results)

- **MAX NUMBER OF PUSH-UPS**

  (2:00 rest, write down your results)

- **MAX TIME HOLDING A PLANK** (write down your results)

  Catch your breath, hydrate and relax. Check your results to see if you should retake the Prep program or move on to Level I.

Knee Push-Up

Knee push-ups are performed exactly as "standard" push-ups (page 62), but instead of your toes touching the ground, your knees will be the point of contact. This eliminates some of the weight of your legs and the smaller angle makes the movement about 15 to 25 percent easier.

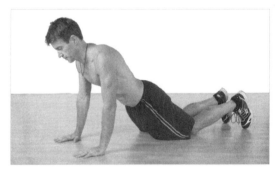

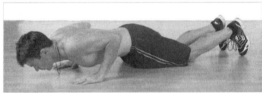

1 Kneel and place your hands on the ground approximately shoulder-width apart. Walk your hands forward until your body forms a straight line from head to knees.

2 Inhale and lower your upper body toward the floor, stopping when your chest is about 3 inches from the floor.

Using your arms, chest, back and core, exhale and push your body back to starting position.

Wall Push-Up

This is easier than all floor push-ups, including those done from the knees.

1 Place your hands on a wall about shoulder-width apart and position your feet as far away from the wall as you feel comfortable. The farther your feet are from the wall, the harder the move will become. Engage your core to keep your back straight and your body in a straight line from head to feet; don't lean your head forward.

2 Inhale as you lower your entire body toward the wall, stopping before your head touches.

Exhale and, using your chest and arms, push your body away from the wall back to starting position.

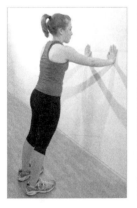

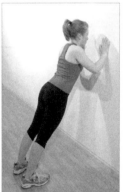

Assisted Pull-Up

If you can't support the weight of your entire body, the best way to learn how to do pull-ups is to get assistance from a spotter or trainer, an exercise band or chair, or use an assisted pull-up machine. Assisted pull-up machines are effective for learning the movement, but don't let the platform become a crutch. If you plan on starting with an assisted machine, make sure you have goals to kick the habit after a short amount of time. A good idea is to decrease the supporting weight every workout by 5 pounds to gradually remove the urge to get lazy. Safety note: *Before using any assisting equipment, make sure any object you use can support your weight and is stable—don't put your safety at risk. If using an exercise band, choose a band based on its pounds of tension ratio; the higher the "weight" of the band, the more assistance it will provide.*

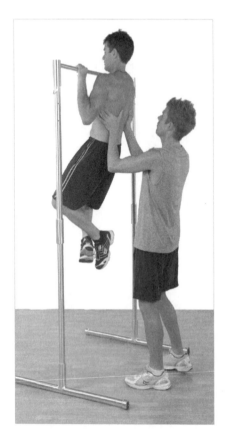

WITH A SPOTTER: Your spotter should place his hands on your shoulder blades (a really good one will even help you squeeze your shoulder blades together at the start of the move) and provide smooth assistance upward and downward in relation to the bar. Never assist by holding someone's feet—if your hands slip off the bar, you'll head toward the floor face-first.

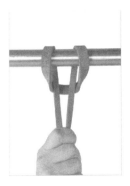

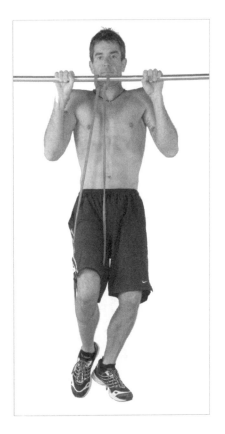

WITH A BAND: Loop the band over the bar and rest your knee on the lower loop. Make sure you're stable and the band will not slip before you begin.

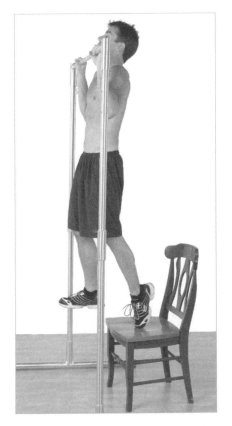

WITH A CHAIR (OR STOOL): Place a stable chair or stool close enough to the bar that you can place your feet on it if necessary to complete a move.

Australian Pull-Up

The Australian pull-up gets its name because you hang "down under" the bar. It's a great way to strengthen the muscles of your upper back, arms and chest while still keeping your feet on the ground. This is much easier than a traditional pull-up because you're not lifting your entire bodyweight. I've done this exercise with lower bars at a playground or with a broom handle placed on the back of two chairs, but I recommend using a Smith machine at a gym with the bar lowered 36" off the floor. Make sure there's enough room for you to extend your arms fully while keeping your upper back off the floor.

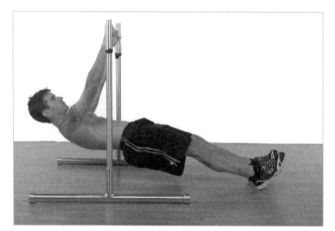

1 Lying face up, extend your feet directly in front of you with the back of your heels in contact with the floor. The bar should be positioned slightly above your chest. Reach up and grab the bar; tighten your core so your spine is erect and your body is in a perfect line from head to heels.

2 Engaging the large broad muscles of your upper back and squeezing your shoulder blades together, pull yourself up and touch your chest to the bar.

Slowly return to starting position.

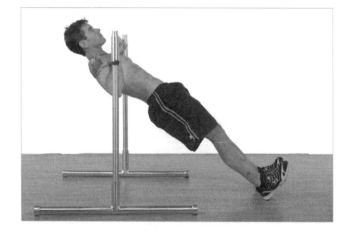

Half Squat

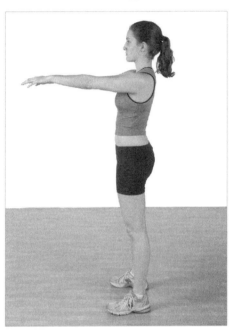

1 Stand with your feet slightly wider than shoulder width and hands extended parallel to the ground in front of you.

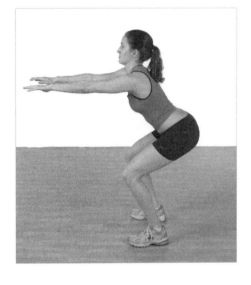

2 Keeping your arms extended in front of you for balance, sit back with your hips and then bend your knees, descending until your upper legs are at a 45° angle to your lower legs.

Return to starting position.

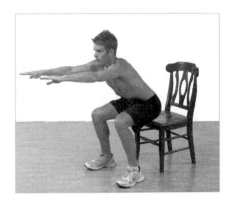

CHAIR VARIATION: Place a chair or bench behind you and perform a proper-form squat, stopping when your behind just barely touches the bench then returning to starting position.

Index

Acknowledgments

Thank you to Jason Warner for helping me create the programs in this book and being a great source of support and inspiration—even from the other side of the world. Residing in Murray Bridge, Australia, Jason created and wrote the games in this book based on the workouts we developed in Scottsdale, Arizona, from 2008–2010. Without Jason's friendship, guidance and commitment to *7 Weeks to Getting Ripped*, this book and programs wouldn't have existed.

Special thanks to Steve Speirs, Lewis Elliot and Corey Irwin for their contributions; to Mike DeAngelo for the continued support and encouragement he has provided for my writing, training and athletics; to Kristen and Vivi for all the love and understanding as well as dealing with me constantly being on my laptop or out training; and to my parents and brother for their unwavering support of their little Booey.

About the Author

Brett Stewart is a National Council for Certified Personal Trainers (NCCPT)–certified personal trainer, a running and triathlon coach, and an endurance athlete who currently 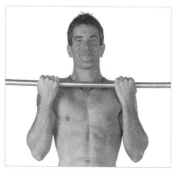 resides in Phoenix, Arizona. An avid multisport athlete and Ironman finisher, Brett has raced dozens of triathlons, multiple marathons and even a few ultra-marathons. He is constantly looking for new fitness challenges and developing new workouts and routines for himself, his friends and his clients. A proud husband and father, Brett is the author of *7 Weeks to 50 Pull-Ups* and can be contacted at 7weekstogettingripped.com.